Fast Facts for the MEDICAL–SURGICAL NURSE: *Clinical Orientation in a Nutshell,* Ciocco

Fast Facts for the LONG-TERM CARE NURSE: *A Guide for Nurses in Nursing Homes and Assisted Living Settings,* Eliopoulos

Fast Facts for the RADIOLOGY NURSE: *An Orientation and Nursing Care Guide in a Nutshell,* Grossman

Fast Facts on ADOLESCENT HEALTH FOR NURSING AND HEALTH PROFESSIONALS: *A Care Guide in a Nutshell,* Herrman

Fast Facts for the ONCOLOGY NURSE: *Oncology Nursing Orientation in a Nutshell,* Lucas

Fast Facts for STROKE CARE NURSING: *An Expert Guide in a Nutshell,* Morrison

Fast Facts for the PEDIATRIC NURSE: *An Orientation Guide in a Nutshell,* Rupert, Young

Visit www.springerpub.com to order.

FAST FACTS FOR
THE NEONATAL NURSE

Michele R. Davidson, PhD, CNM, CFN, RN, CPS, is associate professor of nursing and serves as the coordinator of the Nursing PhD Program at George Mason University in Fairfax, Virginia. Dr. Davidson is a certified nurse midwife (CNM) and a certified forensic nurse (CFN) and has a special interest in high-risk obstetrics and women's mental health issues, including postpartum depression and psychosis.

Dr. Davidson has published over 50 papers, contributed more than 21 chapters to other authors' textbooks, and published an additional 23 textbooks that she has cowritten, including the international bestseller, *Old's Maternal–Newborn Nursing and Women's Health Care Across the Lifespan* (10th ed.), which has been translated into nine languages and used throughout the world. Dr. Davidson recently published *A Nurse's Guide to Women's Mental Health Care,* which earned an *American Journal of Nursing* Book Award in 2012 in the category of psychiatric mental health nursing.

In 2002, Dr. Davidson established the Smith Island Foundation to provide rural health care education, screening programs, and children's programs to a small island community in the Chesapeake Bay. She subsequently developed an immersion clinical practicum for students to participate in rural community health on Smith Island. She is also the author of the children's book *Stowaways to Smith Island.*

FAST FACTS FOR THE NEONATAL NURSE

A Nursing Orientation and Care Guide in a Nutshell

Michele R. Davidson, PhD, CNM, CFN, RN, CPS

SPRINGER / PUBLISHING COMPANY
NEW YORK

Springer Publishing Company, LLC
11 West 42nd Street
New York, NY 10036
www.springerpub.com

Acquisitions Editor: Elizabeth Nieginski
Composition: S4Carlisle Publishing Services

ISBN: 978-0-8261-6882-5
e-book ISBN: 978-0-8261-6883-2

15 16 17 18 / 5 4 3 2

The author and the publisher of this Work have made every effort to use sources believed to be reliable to provide information that is accurate and compatible with the standards generally accepted at the time of publication. Because medical science is continually advancing, our knowledge base continues to expand. Therefore, as new information becomes available, changes in procedures become necessary. We recommend that the reader always consult current research and specific institutional policies before performing any clinical procedure. The author and publisher shall not be liable for any special, consequential, or exemplary damages resulting, in whole or in part, from the readers' use of, or reliance on, the information contained in this book. The publisher has no responsibility for the persistence or accuracy of URLs for external or third-party Internet websites referred to in this publication and does not guarantee that any content on such websites is, or will remain, accurate or appropriate.

Library of Congress Cataloging-in-Publication Data

Davidson, Michele R., author.
  Fast facts for the neonatal nurse : a nursing orientation and care guide in a nutshell / Michele R. Davidson.
      p. ; cm. — (Fast facts)
  Includes bibliographical references and index.
  ISBN-13: 978-0-8261-6882-5
  ISBN-10: 0-8261-6882-5
  ISBN-13: 978-0-8261-6883-2 (e-book)
  I. Title. II. Series: Fast facts (Springer Publishing Company)
  [DNLM: 1. Neonatal Nursing—methods. 2. Infant, Newborn, Diseases—nursing.
3. Perinatal Care—methods. WY 157.3]
  RJ253
  618.92'01—dc23
                                    2014000284

Special discounts on bulk quantities of our books are available to corporations, professional associations, pharmaceutical companies, health care organizations, and other qualifying groups. If you are interested in a custom book, including chapters from more than one of our titles, we can provide that service as well.

For details, please contact:
Special Sales Department, Springer Publishing Company, LLC
11 West 42nd Street, 15th Floor, New York, NY 10036-8002
Phone: 877-687-7476 or 212-431-4370; Fax: 212-941-7842
E-mail: sales@springerpub.com

Printed in the United States of America by Gasch Printing.

For my son,
Grant McPhee Davidson.
My sweet boy, whose very existence is a miracle and blessing
that inspires hope and inspiration to all who cross his path.
His journey in life has not been, and will not be, easy, but he
continually shows others how to transform the impossible into
possibilities. He brings pure joy, determination, and love into the
world and is a ray of sunshine for all who meet him.

Contents

Appendices

Preface

This book provides a basic reference for nurses caring for newborns and high-risk newborns as well as care considerations for families. Nurses continue to function as valued members of a collaborative health care team, play a primary role in the assessment and care of the newborn, and provide education for new parents regarding the newborn's needs. Families experience dramatic transformations as roles develop and change during the newborn period, and rely on the knowledge, support, and encouragement of the nurse to learn to care for their newborn and meet the newborn's most basic needs. In-depth knowledge of the physiological changes of the newborn enables the nurse to detect possible complications that warrant additional assessment. Early identification of risk factors and complications can help ensure that proper newborn evaluation and care are provided when alterations are present.

Advancements in obstetrical care practices have led to advances and options for very premature newborns. Infants who would not have survived if born decades earlier now have far greater chances of survival, though some will have lifelong consequences as a result of birth occurring at early gestational ages. Although most births occur at term and without serious complications, 11.5% of newborns are born prematurely (before 37 completed weeks). Prematurity remains the greatest risk factor for newborn morbidity and mortality. Prematurity is also the leading cause of disabilities in children.

In acute care facilities, it is the nurse who performs the initial newborn assessment and obtains measurements and other assessment data. A thorough knowledge of normal newborn characteristics enables the competent nurse to quickly identify deviations from normal characteristics or potential complications. If an abnormality is identified, it is the nurse's role to notify the clinician and initiate interventions to ensure that stabilization of the newborn is promptly achieved. Most abnormalities, birth defects, or complications are identified during the newborn examination.

The nurse plays an invaluable role in providing education to the family on the proper care of the newborn, including assisting with feedings. Breastfeeding is the preferred method of feeding for all infants, regardless of gestational age. The American Academy of Pediatrics recommends exclusive breastfeeding for the first 6 months of life. Successful and long-term breastfeeding has been noted to be highest in women who receive initial breastfeeding opportunities as soon as possible after birth with assistance from educated nurses who can provide hands-on support. The nurse assists the mother in learning basic provisions for infant feeding and supports the mother's choice of feeding method. Some women will opt not to breastfeed and continue to need guidance and education to ensure proper nutrition for the newborn.

Although the vast majority of infants are born without long-term complications, some newborns experience short-term complications. Although these conditions are short-term in nature, they do require immediate intervention and treatment. Cold stress, hypoglycemia, jaundice, respiratory distress, fluid and electrolyte conditions, and infections are usually not associated with long-term complications if they are identified early and promptly treated. Other complications have ongoing implications that may require more intensive interventions and longer treatment durations, such as prematurity or low birth weight. A small number of infants will be born with conditions that have lifelong implications and may require intensive care or management strategies, such as genetic defects or birth defects.

Although most nurses face ethical dilemmas in practice, the newborn nursery nurse, especially the neonatal intensive care unit nurse, faces these on a regular basis. Infants may be exposed to the mothers' substance abuse and alcohol use in pregnancy, which can have lifelong consequences. Other infants are born on the edge of viability and will require intensely complex decisions to determine the most ethical and compassionate plan of care. Some of these newborns will require emergency procedures, whereas some of these newborns will need transport to obtain life-saving measures. Other newborns will have conditions that are incompatible with life, leaving families facing harrowing issues of death and dying. Any family faced with unexpected birth outcomes, whether they be birth trauma, injury, or previously unidentified disorders, needs extensive support, education, and compassion.

Newborns face multiple vulnerabilities and need specialized care from their caregivers in order to establish normal growth and development and to prevent illness and injury. Nurses must possess excellent communication skills and have knowledge of various procedures and care needs, such as immunizations, proper sleeping positions, fall precautions, and travel recommendations. Nurses give explanations in order to provide comprehensive holistic teaching to families about the initial care for the newborn in the home environment. Ongoing educational needs include the need for newborn examinations, well visits in the infant period, and infant immunizations.

The nurse caring for the newborn also provides a great deal of support and has extensive interaction with the mother and new family. Support for the postpartum family includes identifying potential risk factors, providing referrals for community support groups, and referral to appropriate multidisciplinary providers, such as pediatric providers or lactation support specialists. The nurse also has extensive interactions with the new mother and should perform postpartum depression and mood and anxiety disorders (PMAD) screening. Approximately 20% of new mothers will develop postpartum depression, which can negatively impact the family, including the newborn. Prompt identification and treatment are associated with better outcomes. Care of the mother with a PMAD includes referral to support groups, evaluation by a skilled practitioner for possible pharmacological interventions, and a multidisciplinary approach that includes skilled professionals. Women leaving the hospital without their infant may be at risk for postpartum depression and require additional support related to their individualized circumstances.

There is no greater joy, responsibility, honor, or blessing than to be afforded the opportunity to work with growing families at this amazing time in their expanding lives. Each newborn and family is entirely unique, different and, in some way, utterly amazing. There are those who will pass through a nurse's life and likely be uneventful, and although it is almost sad to say, will likely be, well . . . forgotten, blending in with the many memories that merge together in the days that will eventually create the weeks, months, and years that knit together a nursing career.

Many nurses caring for newborns likely take for granted that sweet baby smell, the smooth skin against your cheek, or the time spent in rockers quieting fussy newborns back to sleep. The daily tasks of life as a nurse can become mundane and typical, but it is my greatest hope that you will embrace each newborn and each new family who comes under your care! For nurses who have their own children, it is likely that, as with your own newborn experience, these days will eventually slip away as you move to a different patient care area, or retirement eventually takes you away, and you will be left reminiscing about your days spent in a nursery rocking chair or feeding a newborn whose mother was sound asleep from a long exhaustive labor. It is quite likely that when that time comes, you will miss those days! It is my hope that actively practicing nurses will enjoy and embrace each and every newborn encounter and that the families will permanently imprint themselves on your heart and soul, providing you with vivid images you can randomly recall. I hope each day continues to instill in you a passion that inspires you to wake up with anticipation, providing you with the reason to continue to care for families during this crucial time period in their lives!

Michele R. Davidson

Acknowledgments

When I was a new graduate nurse, I worked in the postpartum setting and the newborn nursery, and now realize it is the best nursing job there is! Later, I became a certified nurse midwife and was blessed to deliver over a thousand babies and care for thousands more families during that time. Although I loved delivering babies, it is those quiet nights sitting in rocking chairs in a downtown Washington, DC, hospital that I remember most vividly and with the fondest of memories. Throughout that time, I am not sure I was aware of the sacred gift that I had been provided, or that I truly valued the many tremendous experiences encountered, or how much I would miss those snuggly newborns when my career path moved forward. For all the families who shared their precious newborns with me and allowed me to care for their most valued life's treasures, my genuine thanks to you!

Although I rejoiced with many families during perhaps the happiest moments in their lives, I was also privileged to care for newborns facing the greatest of challenges. I have had several newborns die in my arms because their parents couldn't bear to watch them take their last breath. It was many of those families who in their darkest hours shared the most intimate and raw feelings of human heartache that have shaped my philosophy of nursing and of life, and ignited my desire to provide compassionate care to all families as they navigate both the joys and heartaches that often come with having a baby! It is with immense thanks and gratitude that I would like to acknowledge all of those families for providing me with the opportunity to share their joys and tears.

Rebecca Sutter, DNP, CFNP, RN, was a contributor to this book and provided her extensive expertise in newborn assessment and newborn care areas. Becky is a knowledgeable family nurse practitioner who has vast experience in pediatrics, and is a dedicated educator and true friend. Many thanks to her for all her efforts and flawless work on making this book a valuable resource. I have now worked with Elizabeth Nieginski of Springer Publishing on two books. She is a true professional, is extremely supportive, and always has exceptional insight. It is with great appreciation to Elizabeth, who saw this project through from conception to completion, that I give my heartfelt thanks!

Special thanks to my husband, Nathan Davidson, CFNP, who also provided support and expertise in content. His unending support and encouragement are always appreciated and valued. My mom, Geri Lewis, is always my best cheerleader and provides support and encouragement, and lends a hand caring for four active grandchildren to ensure I meet deadlines for my work projects. My father, Harry McPhee, and my "little" brother, Chet McPhee, remain avid supporters of all my work, and their ongoing encouragement is frequent and always appreciated.

My own personal experience with newborns lies with having the absolute joy of bringing home four beautiful babies: Hayden, Chloe, Caroline, and Grant, who have taught me more in their young lives than any professional education or professor could ever provide. My youngest child, Grant, was born at 30 gestational weeks and suffered spastic quadriplegia, giving me direct personal experience with unexpected birth outcomes, which over the years has enabled me to possess a greater understanding of the absolute critical need for empathy, resilience, and hope—critical attributes that families facing these unique challenges truly need. My son is a child who illustrates incredible personal strength, presents with remarkable courage, and never gives up; he chooses to conquer life's struggles with grace, persistence, and determination. He has taught me a great deal about the experiences of unexpected outcomes, birth defects, and losses faced by some parents. He is truly a blessing who has been an inspiration not only to me, but to everyone who has encountered him in his or her life's journey. Our journey and his life are a testament to how one learns from life's greatest challenges and finds the silver lining in what seems like life's gravest events!

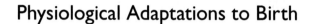

Physiological Adaptations to Birth

The newborn undergoes drastic physiological changes at the time of birth. The neonatal transition period represents the hours following birth when the respiratory and cardiovascular systems stabilize. Other systems may take longer to become fully functioning after birth. The nurse provides ongoing observation and performs frequent assessments during this period to ensure underlying pathological alterations are not present that could interfere with the newborn's successful adaptation to extrauterine life.

During this part of the orientation, the nurse will be able to:

1. Identify normal and abnormal assessment findings in the newborn
2. Describe the changes required by each body system for successful adaptation to extrauterine life
3. Discuss the respiratory and cardiovascular changes that occur during the transition to extrauterine life and during stabilization
4. Describe how various factors affect the newborn's blood values
5. Understand the steps involved in excretion of bilirubin in the newborn and discuss the reasons a newborn may develop jaundice

6. Describe the functional ability of the newborn's liver and gastrointestinal tract
7. Discuss reasons a newborn's kidneys have difficulty maintaining fluid and electrolyte balance
8. List the immunologic responses of the newborn
9. Describe the normal sensory abilities and behavioral states of the newborn

EQUIPMENT

Stethoscope, measuring tape, scale, thermometer.

RESPIRATORY SYSTEM

Physiology of the Respiratory System

- The development of the respiratory system in utero begins with differentiation of structures into pulmonary, vascular, and lymphatic structures.
- Fetal breathing movements, in utero practice respiratory movements, begin by 17 to 20 weeks.
- Beginning at 20 weeks, alveolar ducts begin to develop.
- By 24 to 28 weeks, alveoli differentiate into type I cells, which aid in gas exchange, and type II cells, which produce and store surfactant.
- At 28 to 32 weeks, surfactant production significantly increases, which aids in the lungs' ability to expand and is vital during extrauterine respiration.

Physiological Adaptations Following Birth

- Initiation of neonatal breathing at birth
  - Lung fluid production decreases 24 to 26 hours prior to birth.
  - Lung expansion occurs at the time of birth.
  - Increase in pulmonary circulation occurs.

- Mechanical stimuli
  - Fetal gasp occurs during expulsion and is initiated by a central nervous system trigger in response to the sudden change in pressure and temperature.
  - Fetal chest compression and chest recoils occur during expulsion
  - With neonatal exhalation and crying against a partially closed glottis, positive intrathoracic pressure occurs.
  - Fluid is absorbed into the lymphatic system and capillaries as lung expansion occurs.
- Chemical stimuli
  - Transitory asphyxia occurs due to:
    - Increase in PCO_2
    - Decreases in pH and PO_2
    - Stimulation of the aortic and carotid chemoreceptors triggers the respiratory system in the medulla.
    - Prostaglandin levels drop when the cord is cut.
- Other stimuli
  - Changes in temperature stimulate skin sensors and rhythmic respirations occur.
  - Environmental components include tactile, auditory, visual, and pain stimuli.

Indicators of Initial Normal Functioning

- Respiratory rate 30 to 60 breaths/minute
- Diaphragmatic breathing
- Initially shallow
- Irregular in depth and rhythm

FAST FACTS in a NUTSHELL

Newborns born via cesarean birth may have an increased amount of fluid in their lungs and need observation for neonatal transition, and require additional bulb suctioning.

Indicators of Abnormal Functioning

- Respiratory rate less than 30 or greater than 60 breaths/minute
- Irregular depth (persistently shallow) and irregular rhythm
- Nasal flaring
- Chest retractions
- Generalized cyanosis

FAST FACTS in a NUTSHELL

The newborn is an obligatory nose breather and any obstruction can lead to respiratory distress; it is essential that the nurse monitor for any signs of distress.

CARDIOVASCULAR SYSTEM

Physiology of the Cardiovascular System

- Cardiovascular development begins to occur within 3 weeks of the last menstrual period (LMP), when circulation begins and the structure of the heart begins to form.
- By 4 weeks, the tubular heart beats, beginning at 28 days (post-LMP), and circulation to the fetus and placenta occurs, although detection of the fetal heart rate typically does not occur until 6 to 7 weeks.
- Atrial division occurs at 5 weeks, and the chambers are clearly defined by 6 weeks.
- By 8 weeks, the heart is fully formed and functioning.

Physiological Adaptations Following Birth

- The initial breath at birth decreases pulmonary vascular resistance, increasing blood flow to the lungs.
- Blood returning from the pulmonary veins increases pressure in the right atrium.

- When the umbilical cord is clamped, umbilical venous blood flow stops completely, dropping pressure in the right atrium and increasing systemic vascular resistance.
- Complete transition from fetal circulation to neonatal cardiopulmonary adaptation involves multiple processes (Table 1.1).

TABLE 1.1 Physiological Cardiac Changes From Fetal to Newborn Circulatory System

Physiological Shift in Cardiac Functioning	Physiological Process That Occurs With Change
Increased aortic pressure	Umbilical cord clamping reduces the intravascular space and halts perfusion to the umbilical cord
Decreased venous pressure	Aortic blood flow increases, which accommodates the systemic circulatory needs Blood flow to the inferior vena cava decreases Decreased right atrial pressure occurs Small reduction in venous circulation occurs
Increased systemic pressure	Increase in systemic pressure with circulation no longer needed for the placenta
Decreased pulmonary artery pressure	Lung expansion increases pulmonary circulation as the pulmonary blood vessels dilate, which decreases pulmonary artery resistance Systemic vascular pressure increases to increase systemic perfusion
Closure of foramen ovale	Closure occurs with a shift in the arterial pressure, which stops the shunting of blood between atria Right atrial pressure drops in response to decreasing vascular resistance and increased pulmonary blood flow Functional closure of the foramen ovale occurs after birth at 1–2 hours of age; however, complete closure does not occur until approximately 30 months During crying, hypothermia, cold stress, hypoxia, or acidosis, the foramen ovale could reopen, causing a right-to-left shunt to occur

(continued)

TABLE 1.1 Physiological Cardiac Changes From Fetal to Newborn Circulatory System (*continued*)

Physiological Shift in Cardiac Functioning	Physiological Process That Occurs With Change
Closure of the ductus arteriosus	Pulmonary vascular pressure increases pulmonary blood flow by reversing the blood flow through the ductus arteriosus
	Increased levels of oxygen cause the ductus arteriosus to constrict
	Functional closure occurs 10–15 hours after birth, with complete closure occurring by 4 weeks
Closure of the ductus venosus	Mechanical pressures occur when the umbilical cord is clamped, blood is redistributed, and cardiac output increases, resulting in blood flow to the liver
	Functional closure occurs within 2 months

Indicators of Initial Normal Functioning

- Initial cardiac rate is 110 to 180 beats per minute (bpm) but can be as high as 180 due to initial crying effort.
- Resting heart rate between 110 and 160 bpm
- During certain activity periods, bpm can vary
  - Deep sleep state can be as low as 80 to 100 bpm
  - Active awake state can be up to 180 bpm
- Regular rhythm and rate
- Peripheral pulses should be palpable and bilaterally equal, although pedal pulses may be difficult to palpate.
- Capillary refill time is 2 to 3 seconds.
- Blood pressure (BP) tends to be higher immediately after birth and then decreases by around 3 hours of age. It rises and stabilizes within 4 to 7 days to approximate the initial level reached immediately after birth. The average mean BP is 42 to 60 mmHg in the resting full-term newborn over 3 kg.
- Heart murmurs may be present as the circulation transfers from a fetal to neonatal state and are usually due to the incomplete closure of the ductus arteriosus or foramen ovale.

Indicators of Initial Abnormal Functioning

- Cardiac rates less than 110 or above 180 bpm
- Heart rate less than 90 bpm that does not increase with stimulation (heart block)
- Irregular rate and rhythm
- Reduction in upper extremity pulses (poor cardiac output or peripheral vasoconstriction)
- Absence of pedal pulses (poor cardiac output or peripheral vasoconstriction)
- Prolonged capillary refill time of greater than 4 seconds
- Cyanosis
  - Cyanosis is momentarily relieved by crying (choanal atresia)

Physiology of the Hematological System

- During fetal development, rudimentary blood moves through primitive vessels connecting to the yolk sac and chorionic membranes at 7 gestational weeks.
- The arterial system develops mainly from the aortic arches.
- The venous system emerges from three bilateral veins and is completed by the eighth gestational week.

Physiological Adaptations Following Birth

- Increase in catecholamines results in increased cardiac output required for maintaining increased metabolic oxygen needs related to thermogenesis, breathing, and feeding demands.
- Fetal right-sided dominance switches to left-sided dominance by 3 to 6 months of age.
- Fetal hemoglobin (HgF) is replaced with adult hemoglobin (HgA) by 6 months of age. The hemoglobin levels decline during the first 2 months of life, leading to a phenomenon known as physiological anemia of the newborn. The lowest hemoglobin level occurs around 3 months of age and is called the physiologic nadir.

Normal Newborn Laboratory Values

- Red blood cell (RBC) production and survival are lower in the newborn than in adults. The average neonatal RBC has a life span of 60 to 80 days (two thirds the life span of adult RBCs).
- Normal blood volume ranges from 80 to 90 mL/kg
- White blood cell (WBC) count ranging from 10,000 to 30,000/mm^3 with polymorphonuclear leukocyte (PMN) predominance
- Iron stores will be used to produce new RBCs, which means most infants will require supplemental iron to maintain adequate iron stores.
  - By the sixth month, bone marrow has become the chief site of blood formation.
- Leukocytosis is a normal finding due to the stress of birth and the subsequent increased production of neutrophils during the first few days of life. Neutrophils then decrease by around 2 weeks of age.
- Blood volume varies based on the amount of placental volume received during delivery. It can be altered by delayed cord clamping, gestational age, prenatal or perinatal hemorrhage, and the site of lab draw on the newborn.
- Electrolyte values change based on the age of the newborn (Table 1.2).

FAST FACTS in a NUTSHELL

It is always advisable to keep in mind the reference ranges from your own laboratory.

- Glucose 40 to 60 mg/dL for first 24 hours, then 50 to 90 mg/dL
  - Low blood sugar of 40 to 45 mg/dL requires treatment.

FAST FACTS in a NUTSHELL

Hemoglobin levels in the newborn fall primarily due to a decrease in red blood cell mass rather than from the increasing plasma volume, causing a dilution.

TABLE 1.2 Blood Electrolyte Values for Term Infants

Value	Cord	1–12 hr	12–24 hr	24–48 hr	48–72 hr	> 3 days
Sodium (mEq/L)	147 (126–166)	143 (124–156)	145 (132–159)	148 (134–160)	149 (139–162)	—
Potassium (mEq/L)	7.8 (5.6–12)	6.4 (5.3–7.3)	6.3 (5.3–8.9)	6.0 (5.2–7.3)	5.9 (5.0–7.7)	—
Chloride (mEq/L)	103 (98–110)	101 (80–111)	103 (87–114)	102 (92–114)	103 (93–112)	—
Calcium (mmol/L)	2.33 (2.1–2.8)	2.1 (1.8–2.3)	1.95 (1.7–2.4)	2.0 (1.5–2.5)	1.98 (1.5–2.4)	—
Calcium (mmol/24 hours)	—	1.05–1.37	1.05–1.37	1.05–1.37	1.10–1.44	1.20–1.48
Phosphate (mmol/L)	1.8 (1.2–2.6)	1.97 (1.1–2.8)	1.84 (0.9–2.6)	1.91 (1.0–2.8)	1.87 (0.9–2.5)	—
Magnesium (mmol/L)	—	—	0.72–1.00	—	0.81–1.05	0.78–1.02
Urea (mmol/L)	10.4 (7.5–14.3)	9.6 (2.9–12.1)	11.8 (3.2–22.5)	11.4 (4.6–27.5)	11.1 (5.4–24.3)	—
Creatinine (mmol/L)	—	—	—	0.04–0.11	—	0.01–0.09
C-reactive protein (mg/L)	<7	<7	<7	<7	<7	<7
Lactate (mmol/L)	1.5–4.5	0.9–2.7	0.8–1.2	—	—	0.5–1.4
Albumin (g/L)	28–43	28–43	28–43	28–43	28–43	30–43
Alkaline phosphatase (IU/L)	28–300	28–300	28–300	28–300	28–300	28–300
Thyroid-stimulating hormone	—	—	3.0–120	3.0–30	—	0.3–10
Cortisol (nmol/L)	200–700	200–700	200–700	—	—	—

(continued)

TABLE 1.2 Blood Electrolyte Values for Term Infants (continued)

Value	Cord	1–12 hr	12–24 hr	24–48 hr	48–72 hr	> 3 days
17-hydroxyprogesterone (nmol/L)	—	—	—	—	0.7–12.4	0.7–12.4
Hemoglobin (g/L)	168	—	184	—	178	170
Hematocrit (%)	53	—	58	—	55	54
Mean corpuscular volume	107	—	108	—	99	98
Reticulocytes (%)	3–7	—	3–7	—	1–3	0–1
White cell count × 10⁹/L	18.1 (9–30)	22.8 (13–38)	18.9 (9.4–34)	—	—	12.2 (5–21)
Neutrophils × 10⁹/L	11.1 (6–26)	15.5 (6–28)	11.5 (5–21)	—	—	5.5 (1.5–10)
Lymphocytes × 10⁹/L	5.5 (2–11)	5.5 (2–11)	5.8 (2–11.5)	—	—	5.0 (2–17)
Monocytes × 10⁹/L	1.1	1.2	1.1	—	—	1.1
Eosinophils × 10⁹/L	0.4	0.5	0.5	—	—	0.5
Platelets (10³/mm³)	150–350	150–350	150–350	150–350	150–350	150–350
Prothrombin time (sec)	—	11–14	11–14	11–14	11–14	11–14
Activated partial thromboplastin time (sec)	—	23–35	23–35	23–35	23–35	23–35

- Vitamin K-dependent clotting factors (II XII, IX, X) become active.

===============================*FAST FACTS in a NUTSHELL*

The initial administration of a vitamin K injection protects against prolonged bleeding until the newborn liver begins to function adequately and establishes normal clotting factors.

HEPATIC SYSTEM

Physiology of the Hepatic System

- Human liver development begins during the third week of gestation; however, it is not fully mature until around 15 years of age. It reaches its largest relative size, about 10% of fetal weight, around the ninth week gestation and is about 5% of body weight in the healthy full-term neonate.

Physiological Adaptations Following Birth

The newborn's liver plays a vital role in the following processes:

- Iron storage for new RBC production
  - Prenatally, if the mother's iron intake has been adequate, there is enough iron stored to last 5 months. At around 6 months of age, food containing iron and/or iron supplements must be added to the infant's diet.
- Coagulation
  - The absence of normal flora needed to synthesize vitamin K results in low levels of vitamin K and creates a transient blood coagulation alteration between the second and fifth days after birth.

- Carbohydrate metabolism
  - The newborn cord blood glucose level is 15 mg/dL lower than maternal blood glucose. The newborn's carbohydrate reserve is relatively low, and during the first 2 hours of life the serum blood glucose level declines and then begins to rise, reaching a steady state by about 3 hours. If the fetus experiences hypoxia or stress, the glycogen stores are used and may be depleted. Glucose is the main source of energy in the first 4 to 6 hours of life.
- Conjugation of bilirubin
  - Conjugation is the conversion of bilirubin from the yellow fat-soluble, unconjugated/indirect form into a water-soluble, excretable/direct form.
    - Unconjugated bilirubin (fat soluble) is a potential toxin that is not an excretable form of bilirubin and must be conjugated (made water soluble) in order to be excreted from the body.
  - Unconjugated bilirubin is a breakdown product derived from the heme portion of hemoglobin that is released from destroyed RBCs.
  - Physiological jaundice: occurs after the first 24 hours of life.
    - Physiological hyperbilirubinemia is a buildup of bilirubin due to the normal hemolysis of red blood cells that were needed for fetal circulation before birth and discarded afterward. The imbalance of an immature liver and an overabundance of bilirubin to process allows the yellow pigment from hemolyzed red cells to accumulate in the blood and give the skin and sclera the yellow tone we call *jaundice*.
    - About 50% of all infants exhibit signs of jaundice in the 2 to 3 days after birth due to decreased glucuronyl transferase.
  - Pathological jaundice occurs before 24 hours of life.
    - Pathological hyperbilirubinemia is related to a condition other than normal newborn bilirubin being processed slowly by an immature liver. Such

conditions include an incompatibility between the baby's and the mother's blood types, incompatibility of additional blood factors, or liver problems. There is actual pathology involved that might require more aggressive and lengthier intervention than physiological bilirubin problems.

=== *FAST FACTS in a NUTSHELL*

In utero, the fetus lives in a state of relative hypoxia, with a PaO_2 of approximately 35 mmHg, compared to 80 mmHg for a healthy child or adult. To maximize the oxygen-carrying capacity of the blood, the fetus produces more RBCs, with a hematocrit level up to 60 being normal.

At birth, the newborn's PaO_2 is increased, thus the excess RBCs are no longer needed for oxygen-carrying capacity, and they begin to break down. This is a normal, physiologic change that occurs at birth. The breakdown of these RBCs releases bilirubin into the bloodstream.

If something causes an excessive number of RBCs to break down (such as ABO or Rh incompatibility, birth trauma, or infection) or impairs the baby's ability to pass bilirubin out of the gastrointestinal tract (nothing orally [NPO], delayed stooling, or meconium ileus), the bilirubin level rises. Bilirubin levels at birth are about 3 mg/dL and should not exceed 12 mg.

=== *FAST FACTS in a NUTSHELL*

Nursing care should include keeping the newborn well hydrated and promoting early and frequent elimination. Early feedings tend to keep bilirubin levels down by stimulating intestinal activity, thus removing the contents and not allowing reabsorption.

GASTROINTESTINAL SYSTEM

Physiology of the Gastrointestinal System

- In utero, fetal swallowing, gastric emptying, and intestinal peristalsis occur. By the end of gestation, peristalsis is much more active in preparation for extrauterine life. Fetal peristalsis is also stimulated by anoxia, and low oxygen states in utero (postterm, placental insufficiency, fetal stress, umbilical cord compromise) can cause a premature meconium stool in utero.
- By 36 to 38 weeks of fetal life, the gastrointestinal (GI) system is sufficiently mature to support extrauterine life.

FAST FACTS in a NUTSHELL

Digestion of protein and carbohydrates is adequate; however, fat digestion and absorption are poor due to the absence of adequate pancreatic enzymes.

Physiological Adaptations Following Birth

- The newborn's stomach holds about 50 to 60 cc and can pass meconium 24 to 48 hours after birth.
- Permeability—The newborn's intestines lack the protective mucosal barrier that helps seal off the intestines, decreasing the risk of both bacteria and potential allergens permeating through the intestine into the bloodstream.
- Digestive enzymes—The newborn pancreas does not produce the enzymes, such as amylase, needed to digest complex carbohydrates or starches until around age 3 months. Newborns also produce less lipase during the first year of life.
- The lower esophageal sphincter is still immature and therefore opens more easily than it will later in life. This allows a small amount of food to reflux up. Infants who fail to gain weight due to a large amount of reflux should be further evaluated for gastroesophageal reflux disease.

Indicators of Initial Normal Functioning

- There is a normal physiologic weight loss in the newborn of around 6% to 10% (loss of body water) due to:
  - Diuresis
  - Expulsion of meconium
  - Withholding of water and calories
- The newborn should gain between .5 to 1 ounce per day, double its birth weight by 5 to 6 months of age, and triple birth weight by 1 year of age.
- The normal newborn's pattern of elimination
  - **Stools**—Meconium is stool that contains epithelial cells, bile, and amniotic fluid. In 90% of normal newborns, meconium stools occur within 24 hours of life. This is a black, tarry stool that will transition to brownish green. Transitional stools are part meconium and part fecal stool from digestion of milk. Formula-fed infants will pass two to three bright-yellow stools per day that may appear "seedy" and may have a strong odor, depending on the type of formula. Breastfed infants will pass several small light-yellow stools per day with little or no odor. Formula-fed infants' bowel movements (BMs) will be the consistency of toothpaste, whereas breastfed infants' BMs will remain quite loose as there is little that is not digested. A newborn who does not pass meconium within 24 to 48 hours of birth should be examined for the possibility of imperforate anus, meconium ileus, bowel obstruction, or cystic fibrosis.

URINARY SYSTEM

Physiology of the Kidneys and Urinary System

- Urine production occurs in utero as early as the fourth month, and there are functioning nephrons by 34 to 36 weeks gestation. The glomerular filtration rate of the newborn's kidney is low. The ability to concentrate and dilute urine is attained by 3 months of age; however, before that, monitoring of fluid therapy to prevent overhydrating or dehydration is necessary.

Physiological Adaptations Following Birth

- Many newborns void immediately after birth and 90% by 24 hours of life. A newborn who has not voided by 48 hours of life should be evaluated for adequacy of fluid intake or urinary/bladder abnormality or dysfunction.
- Normal urine is straw colored and odorless.
- In the first 2 days of life the newborn will void two to six times a day, with a urine output of 15 mg/kg/day. Subsequently, the newborn will void between 6 and 25 times every 24 hours, with a urine output of 25 mg/kg/day.
- Following the initial void the newborn's urine is frequently cloudy, due to mucus and a high specific gravity. Pink-stained urine, called "brick dust spots," will occasionally be seen. These are caused by urates and are harmless. Blood may also be observed on the diapers of female newborns. Pseudomenstruation is related to the maternal withdrawal of hormones.

IMMUNOLOGICAL SYSTEM

Physiology of the Immune System

The newborn's immune system is not initiated until after birth. Due to the newborn's limited inflammatory response, there is a failure to recognize and therefore respond to bacteria. This is why the signs and symptoms of infection in the newborn are often subtle and nonspecific.

Of the three major types of immunoglobulins (IgG, IgA, IgM), only IgG is able to cross the placenta. Newborns have what is termed *passive acquired immunity* against viruses to which the mother had antibodies (diphtheria, poliomyelitis, measles, mumps, varicella, tetanus, rubella, smallpox), as a result of maternal IgG that crossed the placenta. These passive maternal immunoglobulins are primarily transferred during the third trimester of pregnancy; therefore, preterm infants may be more susceptible to infection.

Although newborns are able to produce or mount a response to antigens and begin development of antibodies, their immunity is not as effective as in an older child's. Because of this, it is customary to wait to begin the majority of routine immunizations until 2 months of age, when the infant can develop *active acquired immunity* more efficiently.

════════════════════════════*FAST FACTS in a NUTSHELL*

Active acquired immunity—the mother forms antibodies in response to illness or immunization. *Passive acquired immunity*—transfer of immunoglobulins to the fetus in utero (IgG production begins at 20 weeks gestation) or to the infant via breast milk.

Physiological Adaptations Following Birth

════════════════════════════*FAST FACTS in a NUTSHELL*

There is little immunity to herpes simplex virus (HSV), so caretakers with an active HSV infection need to wear a mask and gloves.

NEUROLOGICAL SYSTEM

Physiology of the Neurological System

- Rapid growth of the fetal brain during the last half of fetal life, with peak near time of birth

Physiological Adaptations Following Birth

Babies move through several transition periods in the first 6 hours after birth as their systems change and stabilize.

First alert period: (15–30 minutes after birth) Baby is alert, respirations irregular, responds vigorously to stimulation

Resting period: (30–120 minutes after birth) Color and vital signs are stabilizing, baby sleeps and is difficult to arouse

Second alert period: (4–8 hours after birth) Awakening, becoming responsive to stimuli again, may have a lot of mucus to clear

• Behavioral States

1. Quiet sleep	Deep sleep, no eye movement, respirations quiet and slower
2. Active sleep	Rapid eye movements, may move extremities or stretch
3. Drowsy	Transitional period, yawns, eyes glazed
4. Quiet alert	Infant able to focus on objects or people, tuned in to environment
5. Active alert	Restless, starting to fuss, faster respirations, more aware of discomfort

The newborn's response to stimuli is simple.

• Senses

Touch	The most significant sense in the newborn for the first few weeks of life.
Vision	Newborns can see objects 8 to 12 inches from their eyes. Newborns are most drawn to faces, particularly the eyes. They are able to follow objects to center of visual field. They prefer yellow and red objects and will regard moving objects and changing light intensity.
Hearing	The newborn will turn toward the sound of a voice and tends to be more alert to a high-pitched voice.
Taste	They are able to discriminate between sweet/nonsweet.
Smell	The newborn's ability to smell increases over the first few days of life. The newborn is able to identify mom's breast milk.

Indicators of Initial Normal Functioning

Newborn or infant reflexes are reflexes that are normal in infants but abnormal in other age groups. Normal newborn reflexes include:

Reflex	Description
Moro	Infant's head is gently lifted and then released suddenly, falling backward for a moment. The normal response is for the baby to have a startled look and arms should move sideways with the palms up and thumbs flexed. The baby may cry for a minute.

Reflex	Description
Suck	Sucks when area around mouth is touched.
Startle	Pulls arms and legs in after hearing a loud noise.
Step	Stepping motions when sole of foot touches hard surface.
Tonic neck (fencing position)	When you move the head of a child who is relaxed and lying on his back to the side, the arm on the side where the head is facing reaches straight away from the body with the hand partly open. The arm on the side away from the face is flexed and the fist is clenched tightly. Turning the baby's face in the other direction reverses the position.
Galant (truncal incurvation)	Occurs when you stroke or tap along the side of the spine while the infant lays on the stomach. The infant will twitch his or her hips toward the touch in a back-and-forth motion.
Grasp	Occurs if you place a finger on the infant's open palm. The hand will close around the finger. Trying to remove the finger causes the grip to tighten.
Rooting	When you stroke the infant's cheek, the infant will turn toward the side that was stroked and begin to make sucking motions.
Parachute	Occurs in slightly older infants; when you hold the child upright and then rotate his body quickly face forward (as if falling), the baby will extend his arms forward.
Blinking	Blinks eyes when the eyes are touched or when a sudden bright light appears.
Cough	Coughs when the airway is stimulated.
Gag	Gags when the throat or back of the mouth is stimulated.
Sneeze	Sneezes when the nose is stimulated.
Yawn	Yawns when the body needs more oxygen.

2

Initial Newborn Procedures

The initial newborn examination is performed imme-diately after birth to detect any gross abnormali-ties and identify issues associated with transition to extrauterine life. Immediately after birth, the nurse performs a test to determine an Apgar score, which indicates how the newborn is adapting and ensures that essential vital functions are operating. The nurse ensures proper temperature regulation and provides a neutral thermal environment for the newborn. An assessment is also performed to determine the infant's gestational age. Gestational age assessment is used to determine whether the newborn has any risk factors related to prematurity. Assessments during the first 24 hours after birth provide essential information and ensure the newborn is appropriately adapting to the new external environment. The nurse conducts mul-tiple procedures during this time period to ensure a smooth transition during the newborn period.

During this part of the orientation, the nurse will be able to:

1. Identify components of the initial newborn examination that is performed during the first hour after birth

2. List the variables assessed in Apgar scoring
3. Discuss interventions for maintaining a neutral thermal environment immediately following birth
4. Describe the importance of a gestational age assessment
5. Define the appropriate intervals for newborn assessments during the first 24 hours after birth
6. Identify critical procedures that should be performed in the first 24 hours after birth

EQUIPMENT

Scale, measuring tape, thermometer, electronic blood pressure monitor, stethoscope, cord clamp, gestational age assessment tool, laboratory monitoring equipment, syringe, medications.

INITIAL NEWBORN EXAMINATION

The initial newborn examination is performed at the time of birth, typically as soon as possible after the newborn has been stabilized but no more than 2 hours after birth. The exam is performed in the birthing room at the maternal bedside unless maternal or newborn complications are present. Initially, the following physical examination is performed:

- General assessment for anomalies or abnormalities
- Presence of any birth defects
- Apgar scoring at 1 minute and 5 minutes
- Respiratory assessment
  - Visual inspection for symmetry
  - Assess for symptoms of respiratory distress (tachypnea, bradypnea, irregular respiratory rate, retractions, nasal flaring, cyanosis)
  - Auscultation of lungs
  - Respiratory rate and rhythm (irregular respirations are normal)

- Cardiac evaluation
  - Heart rate
  - Heart rhythm
  - Presence of abnormalities (murmurs, gallops, clicks, extra heart sounds)
  - Cyanosis
- Vital sign assessment
  - Heart rate of 110 to 160 bpm
  - Respirations of 30 to 60 breaths/minute
  - Temperature 97.5 to 99° F (36.0 to 37.2° C)
  - Blood pressure: 70–50/45–30 mmHg
- Umbilical cord assessment (three vessels with Wharton's jelly covering the cord; bleeding, redness, and signs of infection should not be present; cord clamp placed correctly with no skin pinched in clamp)

NEWBORN RESUSCITATION AT TIME OF BIRTH

Newborn resuscitation is warranted when a normal transition with adequate respirations, heart rate, and normal circulation has not been established. Approximately 10% of newborns will need some resuscitation, with only 1% needing intensive efforts. Initial methods of stabilization include:

- Dry newborn, providing stimulation for initial breath.
- Term infants with vigorous crying and good muscle tone should be placed on mother's chest for stabilization.
- Preterm infants, infants without crying or breathing efforts, or those with poor tone should be placed on radiant warmer.
- Provide warmth under radiant warmer.
- Clear airway only if necessary and position head upright in a sniffing position.

- Assess respirations (a crying newborn has adequate respiration; apnea, gasping, or labored breathing may warrant ventilation).
- Evaluate heart rate simultaneously using the umbilical pulse; rates less than 100 bpm warrant intervention.

Resuscitation Procedure

When neonatal distress occurs, resuscitation measures may be warranted. Initial resuscitation involves:

- Evaluation of airway
- Clear the airway via suctioning as needed.
- If poor respiratory functioning is present, positive pressure ventilation (PPV) with an ambubag is begun at 40 to 60 breaths/minute.
- If heart rate is less than 60 bpm after 30 seconds of PPV, chest compressions are warranted.
- If the heart rate remains less than 60 bpm despite adequate ventilation (usually with endotracheal intubation) and 100% oxygen and chest compressions, administration of epinephrine or volume expansion, or both, may be indicated.
- Buffers, a narcotic antagonist, or vasopressors may be useful after resuscitation, but these are not recommended in the delivery room and are rarely needed.
- Typical resuscitation efforts are maintained for 10 minutes before consideration of termination.

NEUTRAL THERMAL ENVIRONMENT

A neutral thermal environment is one in which the newborn maintains his or her current temperature without using body reserves. Heat production in the neonate is via metabolism and nonshivering thermogenesis. Brown fat, which develops by 28 gestational weeks, insulates the newborn and allows for thermogenesis to take place.

Types of Heat Loss

Evaporation: Heat loss occurs from the respiratory tract and skin

Convection: Heat loss to surrounding cooler air

Conduction: Heat loss to solid objects in contact with the body

Radiation: Heat loss to surrounding cooler objects not in direct contact with body

Infants at Risk for Heat Loss and Hypothermia

- Premature infants
- Infants with sepsis
- Infants with central nervous system injuries or anomalies
- Small-for-gestational-age infants
- Prolonged resuscitation efforts

Interventions to Prevent Heat Loss

Preventing heat loss at the time of birth is essential for normal newborn adaptation. Heat loss prevention is achieved by:

- Prewarming warmer prior to birth
- Evaluating environment for temperature instability
- Immediately drying infant at time of birth with warmed blankets
- Removing wet blankets
- Placing infant skin-to-skin with mother
- Covering infant with warmed blankets
  - Placing hat on newborn head
- Initiating early breastfeeding
- Monitoring temperature by axillary temperature assessment
- If low temperature persists, placing infant under radiant warmer

- Assessing blood glucose level; hypoglycemia often precedes cold stress
- Early feeding if hypoglycemia is present
- Placing infants unable to maintain body temperature in a prewarmed isolette and transferring them to the high-risk nursery or neonatal intensive care unit
- Delaying initial bath until three normal temperature readings have been obtained

FREQUENCY OF NEWBORN EXAMINATIONS IN FIRST 24 HOURS OF LIFE

The initial newborn examination should be performed within 2 hours of birth. A complete nursing assessment should then be performed when the newborn is admitted to the newborn nursery. Vital signs should be monitored every 30 minutes for the first 2 hours after birth. Once initial vital signs are completed and are stabilized, vital sign frequency is per agency policy but typically occurs each shift, usually every 8 to 12 hours. A physical examination by a practitioner should be performed within the first 24 hours of birth and again prior to discharge.

PROMOTION OF PARENT–INFANT ATTACHMENT

Early positive interactions between the parents and newborn help facilitate parent–infant attachment. The nurse can provide the following interventions to aid in the attachment process:

- Place infant skin to skin with parent.
- Encourage early breastfeeding.
- Educate parents on normal newborn characteristics and behaviors.
- Advise parents what to expect in terms of infant behavior and interaction with others.

- Encourage parents to touch newborn.
- Encourage rooming-in and constant contact.
- Assist parents in providing care for the newborn.
- Include siblings and extended family in early interactions with newborn.
- Encourage eye contact.
- Demonstrate swaddling procedure.
- Encourage parents to rock their infants, hold them upright, and talk to their infants.
- Describe normal sleep–wake patterns.

APGAR SCORING

The Apgar score is a screening test that was developed by Dr. Virginia Apgar in 1952 and is now used worldwide to quickly assess the health of an infant 1 minute and 5 minutes after birth (Table 2.1). The 1-minute Apgar score measures the newborn's tolerance of the birth, whereas the 5-minute score assesses how well the newborn is adapting to the external environment.

The Apgar score evaluates the following:

- Heart rate
- Breathing
- Activity and muscle tone
- Reflexes
- Skin color

TABLE 2.1 Apgar Scoring System

Characteristics	Score of 0	Score of 1	Score of 2
Color	Blue or pale over entire body	Acrocyanosis with pink body	Body pink all over, including extremities
Heart rate	Absent	< 100 bpm	> 100 bpm
Reflexes	No response to stimulation	Grimace, weak cry with stimulation	Vigorous crying or pulls away with crying

(continued)

TABLE 2.1 Apgar Scoring System (*continued*)

Characteristics	Score of 0	Score of 1	Score of 2
Activity	None	Some flexion	Flexed arms and legs that resist extension
Respiratory	Absent	Weak, irregular gasping	Strong lusty cry

As indicated previously, the Apgar score is assigned at 1 and 5 minutes after birth. Over 98% of infants have a 5-minute Apgar score of greater than 7. Scores less than 7 indicate that ongoing medical intervention is warranted. Low 5-minute Apgar scores are not necessarily indicative of long-term adverse health outcomes. Low 5-minute scores are most commonly associated with traumatic births, cesarean births, and fluid in the neonate's lungs. If the score remains below 7 at 5 minutes, a 10-minute Apgar score can be given, with continued scores every 5 minutes until 20 minutes of age. Apgar scores of 7 to 10 at 5 minutes are considered normal.

GESTATIONAL AGE ASSESSMENT

Gestational age assessment is important in determining needs and possible risks in the early neonatal period. Multiple gestational age assessment methods are available to evaluate and determine the newborn's gestational age. These tests evaluate the newborn's appearance, skin texture, motor function, and reflexes. The physical maturity portion of the exam should be performed within the first 2 hours of birth. The neuromuscular maturity examination should be completed within 24 hours after birth. The New Ballard Score system was developed in 1991 to screen extremely premature infants.

PHYSICAL MATURITY CHARACTERISTICS

The newborn's physical characteristics are examined. These include:

- Skin—ranges from sticky and red in preterm infants to smooth to cracking or peeling in postmature infants.
- Lanugo (the soft downy hair on a baby's body) is absent in immature babies, appears with maturity, and then disappears again with postmaturity.
- Plantar creases—these creases on the sole of the feet range from absent to covering the entire foot depending on the maturity.
- Breast—the thickness and size of breast tissue and areola (the darkened nipple area) are assessed.
- Eyes and ears—eyes fused or open and amount of cartilage and stiffness of the ear tissue are assessed.
- Genitals, male—presence of testes and appearance of scrotum, from smooth to wrinkled.
- Genitals, female—appearance and size of the clitoris and the labia.

NEUROMUSCULAR MATURITY CHARACTERISTICS

The neuromuscular characteristics used to determine gestational age include:

- Posture—how the baby holds his or her arms and legs
- Square window—how much the baby's hand can be flexed toward the wrist
- Arm recoil—how much the baby's arms "spring back" to a flexed position
- Popliteal angle—how much the baby's knee extends
- Scarf sign—how far the elbow can be moved across the baby's chest
- Heel to ear—how close the baby's foot can be moved to the ear

NEWBORN PROCEDURES

The newborn undergoes a number of procedures during the first hours after birth. Nurses should provide new parents with detailed information on the rationale for the procedure, what the procedure involves, and expected outcomes for each procedure. Some parents may have concerns and fears about some procedures and require reassurance and education from the nursing staff.

Cord Blood Testing

Cord blood testing is done at the time of birth after the umbilical cord is clamped and cut. When cord blood is drawn, another clamp is placed 8 to 10 inches away from the first. The isolated section is then cut and a blood sample is collected into a specimen tube. Cord blood testing is not always performed, but can be done for the following testing purposes:

- Bilirubin levels
- Blood culture (if an infection is suspected)
- Blood gases, to evaluate the oxygen, carbon dioxide, and pH levels
- Blood type and Rh
- Complete blood count
- Glucose levels
- Platelet count

Cord Blood Banking

Cord blood banking is an elective procedure in which the parents opt to have the newborn's cord blood collected and stored. Cord blood contains stem cells that can be used to treat more than 80 diseases, including cancers and blood disorders. Families with a history of rare disorders or cancers may opt to collect cord blood for future use by the child or other family members. Cord blood collection involves a significant cost that is incurred by the family. Some volunteer donation programs are in existence but are typically rare.

Vitamin K Administration

Vitamin K is administered for prevention of hemorrhage in the first few days of life. Due to the absence of gut flora and low prothrombin levels at birth, newborns are at an increased risk for hemorrhage. Vitamin K_1 (AquaMEPHY-TON) is administered via intramuscular injection into the vastus lateralis muscle. The injection is typically given within the first hour after birth.

===== *FAST FACTS in a NUTSHELL*

Vitamin K injections should always be administered prior to a circumcision procedure due to the risk for bleeding.

Erythromycin Gel Administration to Eyes

Prophylactic antibiotic eye treatment is now legally required at the time of birth to prevent transmission of gonorrhea during the birth process. Erythromycin gel is the most commonly used agent to prevent infection. The ointment is administered into the lower conjunctival sac of each eye. The ointment may cause edema, blurred vision, and some discomfort that resolves in 1 to 2 days. Eye treatment should be administered within 1 hour of birth.

Hepatitis B Vaccine

Hepatitis B vaccination is now recommended for all new-borns at the time of birth. Infants should receive the initial immunization in the hospital and complete the series by the age of 12 to 18 months. Infants weighing less than 2,000 grams whose mothers are negative for hepatitis B maternal surface antigen can delay the vaccine until 1 month of age or receive the vaccine at the time of discharge from the hospital. Infants born to mothers with unknown status or a positive hepatitis B surface antigen should receive the vaccine within 12 hours of birth.

Hearing Screening

Newborn hearing loss is one of the most commonly occurring birth defects and affects 3 per 1,000 births. Hearing loss can impede speech, language, social, and cognitive development. Currently, 43 states mandate newborn hearing screening measures. It is estimated that 95% of all newborns in the United States are screened prior to hospital discharge. Screening tests include the auditory brainstem response evaluation or the otoacoustic emission measure.

Failed Newborn Hearing Screenings

Parents should be counseled that a failed test can occur as a result of excessive noise in the room, excessive newborn movement during the test, and, most commonly, from amniotic fluid accumulation in the ears. If an infant fails the initial test, a second test is performed at least 1 week later. Infants who fail the second test should be referred to a pediatric audiologist for more definitive screening.

3

Comprehensive Newborn Exam

Each infant undergoes an initial physical examination in the delivery room immediately after birth to detect gross abnormalities and birth defects and to assess the newborn's transition to extrauterine life. A comprehensive examination is then typically performed within the first 2 hours of birth, once the newborn enters the nursery. The comprehensive examination includes a complete review of the maternal medical and social history, genetic history, prenatal history, the course of the labor and birth, head-to-toe assessment, and weight and measurements of the newborn. The nurse performs the initial assessment in the delivery room and then completes the comprehensive examination. The pediatric care provider is then notified of the infant's status. Any abnormalities identified may warrant prompt intervention or referral for additional assessments from specialty providers.

During this part of the orientation, the nurse will be able to:

1. Identify the appropriate time parameters for performance of the initial newborn evaluation and the comprehensive newborn assessment

2. List the historical information that is pertinent to review prior to performing the newborn examination
3. Describe the normal newborn appearance
4. List the routine measurement data that are obtained during a comprehensive newborn examination
5. Discuss normal skin variations present in newborn infants
6. Compare and contrast normal and abnormal physical characteristics in the newborn
7. Describe components of a newborn behavioral assessment

REVIEW OF HISTORICAL DATA

The comprehensive examination begins with a review of pertinent data, including maternal medical information, genetic factors, prenatal history, and the course of labor and birth events. Certain maternal medical and social factors can have implications for the newborn, including:

- Maternal hypertensive disorders
- Preexisting diabetes
- Coagulation defects
- Infections (hepatitis B, HIV, herpes simplex virus)
- Tobacco, alcohol, or substance use in pregnancy

Genetic Factors

A careful review of familial disease and genetic conditions is important to identify possible genetic conditions that may be present in the newborn. Ideally, parents should have undergone genetic counseling during the prenatal period. Any newborn who has a suspected genetic defect should undergo an evaluation with a genetic specialist and karyotype testing.

Prenatal History

Pregnancy history can provide pertinent data that may impact the newborn. A careful review of the prenatal record is imperative. Any maternal medical conditions, infectious disease exposure during pregnancy, medications used during pregnancy, and pregnancy-related complications should be reported.

Labor and Birth History

The course of the labor and birth can impact the initial newborn transition and may yield long-term implications for the infant. The following factors should be reviewed:

- Length of labor
- Length of rupture of membranes
- Presence of maternal fever
- Presence of nonreassuring fetal status
- Spontaneous or induced labor
- Type of birth (vaginal, cesarean section, operative vaginal birth)
- Length of second stage
- Any birth-related complications (shoulder dystocia, prolonged second stage, nonreassuring fetal status)
- Apgar scores
- Need for resuscitation

WEIGHT AND MEASUREMENTS

Weight and measurements provide initial data that are then used throughout infancy to track growth and development. Background information related to weight and measurements includes:

- Shortly after birth, the newborn is weighed.
- The weight is recorded in both pounds and grams. The average Caucasian infant weighs 3,405 grams (7 pounds 8 ounces). Other races tend to have infants with lower birth weights.
- Infants may lose 10% to 15% of their birth weight during the first few days of life.
- Larger and premature infants often experience greater weight loss. Initial weight loss occurs in the first few days after birth.

- After the first week of life until the age of 6 months, infants typically gain 7 ounces per week. The infant's weight should be plotted on a maturity-and-growth chart.
- Length is obtained by stretching the infant fully and measuring from the top of the head to the heel with the infant in a straightened position.
- The average length for a full-term newborn is 50 centimeters (20 inches), with a range of 48 to 52 cm (18 to 22 inches).
- Infants typically grow 1 inch per month during the first 6 months of life.
- Head circumference is obtained by measuring the prominent portion of the occiput and extending the tape to above the eyebrows to obtain the circumference of the head.
- The circumference of the head should be 2 cm greater than the chest circumference.
- The average head circumference is 32 to 37 centimeters (12.5 to 14.5 inches).
- Molding, caput, and cephalohematomas can alter the measurement.
- Reassessing the measurement at 2 days of age often provides a more accurate measurement.
- Chest circumference is measured by placing the measuring tape over the nipple line in the front and at the lower edge of the scapula in the back.
- The average chest circumference is 32 cm (12.5 inches), with a normal range of 30 to 35 cm (12 to 14 inches).
- Abdominal circumference can also be recorded but in general it is not a standardized measurement.

SKIN

Skin variations are common and vary for many of reasons:

- Newborns typically have a ruddy complexion due to limited brown fat and increased red blood cells in blood vessels that are close to the surface.

- Skin color varies based on ethnicity.
  - Caucasian newborns are typically pinkish in color immediately after birth.
  - African American newborns range from a pale pink with a yellowish or red hue to a reddish-brown color.
  - Asian and Hispanic babies are typically pink in color, rosy red with a yellow hue, or have an olive or yellow skin tone.

Various skin variations are common in newborns. These variations are found in Table 3.1.

HEAD AND NECK

The newborn may have variations in the head directly associated with the birth process.

- The newborn head is often molded and misshaped due to the birth process.
- *Molding* occurs, allowing the cranial bones to change shape and overlap to facilitate vaginal birth.
- Due to variations in head shape after birth, the head circumference measure may not be accurate during the first few days of life.
- The head may be covered by hair, although some infants are born with no hair at all. In general, any variation in normal hair distribution, texture, or quantity can indicate abnormalities in metabolic, genetic, or neurological disorders.
- The head has two fontanels that are open between the cranial bones, which allows for head growth during infancy and early childhood. The fontanels should be assessed during the newborn exam:
  - Anterior fontanel is diamond-shaped and is 3 to 4 cm long and 2 to 3 cm wide, and is located between the frontal and parietal bones. Closure occurs by 18 months.

TABLE 3.1 Skin Variations in Newborns

Skin Variation	Physical Description	Common Conditions Associated With Skin Condition
Acrocyanosis	Bluish coloration in hands and feet	Common in first 6 hours after birth. Can also be associated with circulatory issues and cold stress.
Erythema toxicum	Eruption of lesions around hair follicles that consist of yellow or white pustules or papules with an erythematous base. Also known as newborn rash or flea-bite dermatitis.	None. May be an allergic dermatitis related to clothing.
Forceps marks	Reddened areas, commonly over cheeks or jaw, related to difficult forceps birth	Forceps birth
Harlequin sign	A unilateral color change that develops over one side of the body while the other side remains pale. The dramatic color change is temporary and lasts 1–20 minutes. Multiple recurrent episodes are common.	None known
Jaundice	Yellowish skin color related to increases in bilirubin levels	Prematurity, blood incompatibility, forceps or vacuum birth, hematomas, immature liver function, or oxytocin administration during labor. More common in breastfed infants.
Milia	Exposed sebaceous glands resulting in small raised white spots on the face and nose	None
Mottling	Lace-like patterns of dilated blood vessels that occur as a result of fluctuations in circulation	Cold stress, apnea, sepsis, hypothyroidism

(continued)

TABLE 3.1 Skin Variations in Newborns (continued)

Skin Variation	Physical Description	Common Conditions Associated With Skin Condition
Mongolian spots	Macular areas of bluish-black or gray-blue pigmentation found on the lower back and over the buttocks	More common in African American, Hispanic, and Asian infants
Nevus flammeus (port wine stain)	Capillary angioma below the epidermis with dark red to purple area of dense capillaries that does not change over time	Commonly occurs on the face. Can be a sign of Sturge-Weber syndrome and is associated with seizures and visual issues.
Nevus vasculosus (strawberry mark)	Capillary hemangiomas are collections of capillaries in the dermal and subdermal layers that are raised, clearly defined, and fade over time.	None
Telangiectatic nevi (stork-bite marks)	Pale pink or red spots over the eyelids, nose, lower occipital bone, and back of the neck. Usually resolve by 24 months of age.	None
Vernix caseosa	A whitish cheese-like substance that covers the newborn	More abundant in preterm newborns

- Posterior fontanel is triangle shaped, is 0.5 to 1 cm long, and is located between the parietal and occipital bones. Closure occurs between 8 and 12 weeks. The neck is short, creased, and symmetrical in appearance.
- The neck contains skin folds, although the back of the neck lacks skin folds.
- The thyroid is in midposition but should not be visible on inspection. The shoulders and clavicle are symmetrical, straight, and smooth.

FACE, EYES, NOSE, AND MOUTH

The face, eyes, nose, and mouth should be assessed. The following findings are common:

- The face should be symmetrical with symmetrical movements.
- Asymmetrical movements may indicate facial paralysis.
- The eyes are equally set and parallel to the pinna of the ear.
- The eyes should be checked to ensure equal pupil size, reaction of pupils to light, blink reflex, red retinal reflex, and any presence of eyelid edema, which can occur.
- Subconjuctival hemorrhages can occur and typically resolve in the first month of life.
- Nose midline
- Nares patent
  - If respiratory difficulties are present, assess to ensure nares are patent.
- Nasal breathing with mouth closed
- Mouth pink with moist mucous membranes
- Mouth symmetrical with the hard and soft palates intact
  - Asymmetry of the mouth can be associated with birth trauma and can indicate nerve damage.

- Gums smooth and pink
- Epstein pearls (glistening white spots) may be present.
- Supplementary teeth (precocious teeth) may be present.
- Tongue pink in color with a rough texture, protrusion, proportionate in size to the mouth, and movable in all directions
- Gag and swallowing reflexes should be intact.

═══════════════*FAST FACTS in a NUTSHELL*

Newborns with Down syndrome and other genetic anomalies may have tongues that protrude, with hypotonia being common, giving them an appearance that the tongue is always sticking out. Infants with Down syndrome also have a narrower palate with a higher curve, which may cause breastfeeding difficulties.

CHEST AND LUNGS

The chest and lungs are assessed and normal characteristics or variations are documented:

- The average chest circumference for a newborn is 32.5 cm (12.5 inches), with a range of 30 to 35 cm (12 to 14 inches).
- The chest is wider than it is long and size varies based on gestational weight.
- The sternum is approximately 8 cm long and may appear to protrude slightly.
- The chest should be a cylinder shape and is symmetrical, with pliable ribs and bilateral expansion.
- The lungs should be bilaterally clear to auscultation at rest and with crying.
- The cough reflex develops within 2 to 3 days of birth.

If rales are present, it likely represents normal atelectasis. Intercostal, subcostal, or supraclavicular retractions are indicative of respiratory compromise and warrant additional assessment and intervention.

HEART AND PERIPHERAL PULSES

The cardiovascular system is evaluated by assessing the heart and peripheral pulses.

- The fetal heart lies horizontally with the left border extending to the left midclavicular line and the apex between the fourth and fifth intercostal space.
- The normal newborn heart rate is 100 to 160 bpm but may be as high as 180 bpm.
- The heart produces a characteristic "lub dub" sound.
- Murmurs that sound like a slur or swishing sound may be present.
  - The majority of murmurs are benign and resolve in the newborn period.
- Peripheral pulses are palpated to determine any abnormalities.
- Pulses should be symmetrical and be equal in nature.
  - Abnormalities in peripheral pulses may indicate cardiac defects or hypervolemia and warrant additional assessment.

ABDOMEN

The normal newborn abdominal exam includes assessment of the abdomen and abdominal organs.

- Abdomen protrudes and is cylinder-shaped.
- Bowel sounds should be present within 1 hour of birth in all four quadrants.

- Abdomen should be soft and nondistended.
- Liver can be palpated 1 to 2 cm below the right costal margin.
- Spleen is palpated in the lateral aspect of the left upper quadrant.
- The lower portion of the kidney is palpable 1 to 2 cm above the level of the umbilicus.

═══════════════════════════════ *FAST FACTS in a NUTSHELL*

Kidney palpation may or may not be performed by nursing staff. If the palpation is part of the newborn exam, it should be assessed within 6 hours of birth, prior to the intestines filling with air, which makes palpation more difficult.

UMBILICAL CORD

The umbilical cord should be assessed as closely as possible to the time of birth because drying distorts the vessels, making assessment more difficult.

- Cord should contain three vessels, two arteries, and one vein.
  - Newborns with a missing umbilical artery have a 25% risk of having additional defects, including cardiac, skeletal, intestinal, or renal problems.
- Umbilical cord must be covered in Wharton's jelly.
- No evidence of bleeding, odor, and drainage should be present.
- No umbilical hernia should be noted.
  - Umbilical hernias occur and are more common in African males and low-birth-weight infants. Umbilical hernias do not typically require intervention and often resolve by 24 months.

GENITALIA

Formation of the genitals occurs in the first trimester. The newborn's genital exam provides data important for the gestational age assessment. The newborn's genitals are inspected and any abnormalities are documented and warrant assessment from a specialist. The female genitalia has the following characteristics:

- Female labia majora, labia minora, and clitoris all develop based on gestational age.
  - Full-term females will have the labia majora covering the labia minora and clitoris.
  - Premature female newborns will have more prominent labia minora with the clitoris clearly visible.
- A hymen tag or vaginal tag is sometimes present.
- Pseudomenstruation is common, which is characterized by a whitish blood-tinged discharge occurring as a result of withdrawal of maternal hormones.
- Smegma is a white, cheese-like substance that is often present between the labia.

The male genitalia has the following characteristics:

- Urinary meatus at the tip of the penis
  - Hypospadias occurs when the meatus opening is on the vertical surface of the penis.
- The foreskin should be inspected to ensure it can be retracted properly over the penis.
  - *Phimosis* is a condition in which the foreskin will not adequately retract over the penis and often requires surgical intervention.
- The color and position of the testes are dependent on gestational age.
  - Before 36 weeks, the scrotum is small with few rugae, with the testes in the inguinal canal. By term, the entire scrotum is covered with rugae.
  - At term, a testicle should be palpable in each scrotal sac.

- Each testicle should be palpated separately to confirm it has descended.
  - *Cryptorchidism* is the failure of a testicle to descend and warrants follow-up to prevent long-term complications.
- Hydrocele, which is a collection of fluid in the scrotum, may occur after birth and typically resolves without intervention.

EXTREMITIES

An assessment of the extremities is performed and documented:

- Extremities are inspected and should be symmetrical in size and proportion.
- Arms should be flexible without gross abnormalities, extra digits, webbing, or clubfoot.
- Range-of-motion abnormalities or lack of movement may occur with brachial plexus (partial or complete paralysis of arm related to birth trauma).
- Erb's palsy typically results in upper arm paralysis, in which the arm lies in a limp position and remains motionless.
- Arms should be symmetrical and bend easily with good range of motion.
- Hands should be inspected and the pattern of palmar creases should be documented.
  - A single palmar crease may be indicative of genetic anomalies and may warrant further testing.
- Legs and feet should be bilaterally symmetrical, with the skin folds of the thighs in equal proportion to each other.
- The Barlow maneuver should be performed to detect congenital hip dysplasia.
- Feet are inspected to ensure they are in proper position.
- Observe for presence of clubfoot.

- Positional clubfeet are sometimes present and are most commonly associated with breech position.
- Positional clubfoot is treated with range-of-motion exercises, whereas a true clubfoot will require surgical intervention.

FAST FACTS in a NUTSHELL

To assess for hip dysplasia, the nurse grasps both thighs simultaneously and adducts the thighs, applying gentle pressure in a downward motion. If the femoral head slips out of the acetabulum, dislocation is probable. The Ortolani's maneuver is performed when the infant is at rest, with the knees and thighs flexed at a 90-degree angle. The nurse grasps the thigh with the middle finger over the trochanter and lifts the thigh toward the acetabulum. With gentle abduction, the head is returned to the acetabulum and an audible click is heard if the hip is dislocated.

BACK

The back should be inspected:

- Skin is intact over the entire spine.
- Spine should be straight.
- The base of the spine should be carefully evaluated to ensure a nevus pilosus (hairy nevus) is not present.
  - The presence of a nevus pilosus can be associated with spina bifida.
- Some infants may have a pilonidal dimple, which can also be related to spina bifida and warrant further assessment.

BEHAVIORAL ASSESSMENT

A newborn behavioral assessment scale assesses the newborn's responses to the environment, neurological abilities, and capabilities. The scale includes 28 behavioral and 18 reflex items and is designed to assess the baby's capabilities across different developmental areas and describes how the baby reacts to the new environment. Components to be measured include:

- Habituation
- Orientation to inanimate and animate visual and auditory stimulation
- Motor activity
- Variations in alert states, state changes, and color changes
- Self-quieting abilities
- Social behaviors (cuddling)

═══════════════════════════ *FAST FACTS in a NUTSHELL*

Newborn behaviors vary considerably during the initial 72 hours of birth; therefore, a complete behavioral assessment should not be performed prior to 3 days of life.

4

Newborn Nutrition

Adequate newborn nutrition is essential for human life, and the process of nursing is linked with the formation of a lasting attachment with the caregiver and stimulates psychosocial development. Parents need extensive education in the basics of newborn feeding to ensure adequate growth and development during the first few weeks of life. Breastfeeding is recommended for nearly all newborns; however, some families will opt for formula feeding. Breastfeeding support, encouragement, and initial instruction are components of care that are associated with long-term breastfeeding success. Nurses need to possess knowledge and skills to help new mothers master early breastfeeding.

Infant feeding practice decisions involve a variety of factors, including comfort with breastfeeding, modesty, family values, and cultural norms. Some women will not feel comfortable breastfeeding and will choose formula feeding. These women should be fully supported in their decision making and should receive educational information on proper formula preparation and storage.

Premature infants require special attention and may warrant supplemental feedings. Prematurity and low birth weight put premature infants at risk for poor postnatal growth in the newborn and early-infancy period. Family education should include variations in growth patterns for families with premature infants.

During this part of the orientation, the nurse will be able to:

1. Identify the nutritional components, including vitamins and minerals, that are essential for normal growth and development in the newborn and infant
2. Name nursing interventions that help support successful breastfeeding in the early postpartum period
3. List the benefits of breastfeeding
4. Identify the contraindications for breastfeeding
5. Describe types of commercial formulas that are available for mothers who wish to formula feed
6. Compare and contrast the breast-milk rule of 5's with the formula rules of 1's
7. Identify growth variations that commonly occur in the premature infant

NUTRITIONAL NEEDS OF NEWBORNS

In the first few months of life, the brain grows at a rapid rate and adequate food and nutrition are needed for both physiological and psychological growth and development.

Calories

- In order for the infant to maintain himself or herself and ultimately grow, the caloric needs for the newborn up to 2 months of age are approximately 110 to 120 calories per kilogram of body weight (50 to 55 kcal/pound) every 24 hours (Table 4.1).
- Calorie needs will vary depending on activity level and growth rate.
- Commercial formulas simulate breast milk and get 9% to 12% of calories from protein and 45% to 55% of calories from lactose carbohydrate. The balance of the formula consists of fat, of which about 10% (4% of the calories) consists of linoleic acid.

TABLE 4.1 Energy Expenditure of an Infant	
Resting energy use	40 kcal/kg/day
Minimal activity	2–4 kcal/kg/day
Occasional cold stress	10 kcal/kg/day
Loss of energy from bowel movements	10 kcal/kg/day
Growth	40 kcal/kg/day
Total	100–105 kcal/kg/day

FAST FACTS in a NUTSHELL

An infant who cries frequently and squirms constantly needs more calories.

Protein

Protein is necessary for formation of new cells. The newborn requires around 2.2 g/kg of body weight in protein intake daily. Unaltered cow's milk is not recommended for newborns because it gets 16% of its calories from protein, whereas human milk contains 8%; the protein in cow's milk can be overwhelming to the newborn's kidneys. Additionally, cow's milk is difficult for the newborn to digest.

Fat

Linoleic acid, an essential fatty acid, is necessary for growth and skin integrity in infants and is found in both breast milk and commercial formulas.

Carbohydrate

Lactose is the most easily digested carbohydrate. Carbohydrates are needed to allow protein to be used for building new cells. Additionally, carbohydrates encourage normal water balance and prevent abnormal metabolism of fat. They have been shown to also aid in calcium absorption and improve nitrogen retention.

Fluid

- Neonates are born with an excess of total body water; this is primarily extracellular fluid (ECF).
- Term neonates usually lose between 5% and 10% of their birth weight in the first week of life, and almost all of this weight loss is the excess ECF.
- With a high metabolic rate and immature kidney function that do not fully concentrate urine, the newborn needs to be monitored closely for fluid volume depletion and dehydration.
- Fluid requirements for the newborn are between 150 and 200 mL/kg per 24 hours and should be completely supplied by breastfeeding or formula feeding.

FAST FACTS in a NUTSHELL

Term neonate bodies are 75% water, 40% ECF, and 35% intracellular fluid.

Calcium

Calcium is essential for the infant's bone growth. If a newborn's ability to suck is adequate, and the child is therefore receiving the necessary nutrition, a low calcium level seldom occurs.

Iron

Term infants of a mother who had adequate iron intake during pregnancy will be born with iron stores lasting for 3 months, which is when the newborn begins to produce hemoglobin. Most mothers do not get adequate iron in their diet and therefore a supplement is recommended for formula-fed infants for 1 year. Most commercially prepared formulas have iron supplementation for this reason. Breast-fed infants receive an adequate iron supply.

Fluoride

Teeth grow into their primary form during pregnancy, so it is important for mothers to drink fluoridated water during and after pregnancy to supply the baby. Fluoride is also contained in most commercially prepared formulas. A fluoride supplement of 0.25 mg/day may be given to infants starting at 6 months of age. However, it should be noted that this can be detrimental or stain teeth.

Vitamins

Vitamins are not routinely needed or necessary for bottle-fed infants because vitamins A, C, and D are available to the infant in commercial formulas. Vitamins are naturally found in breast milk; however, breast-fed newborns may need to be exposed to sunlight to receive adequate vitamin D (or the mother can take 400 U daily). Vitamins are not routinely given to infants younger than 6 months of age.

Breastfeeding

Breastfeeding is clearly the preferred feeding method for the newborn and is the ideal nutrition source for infants during the first year of life and beyond. Evidence has shown breast-feeding to have immediate as well as long-term health benefits.

FAST FACTS in a NUTSHELL

The American Academy of Pediatrics recommends *exclusive* breastfeeding for the first 6 months. The World Health Organization recommends breastfeeding for 2 or more years.

NURSING INTERVENTIONS TO SUPPORT BREASTFEEDING

Nurses play a major role in educating new parents about the benefits and management of breastfeeding. Key interventions include:

- Helping to initiate breastfeeding within 30 minutes of birth
- Assisting the new mother with breastfeeding and ensuring lactation, even if the infant must be separated from the mother
- Advocating against supplemental feedings other than breast milk unless medically indicated
- Avoiding providing pacifiers to breastfeeding infants until breastfeeding has been well established
- Advocating for mother/infant rooming-in
- Encouraging breastfeeding on demand
- Fostering the establishment of breastfeeding support groups and referring mothers to lactation consultants as needed

PHYSIOLOGY OF BREAST MILK PRODUCTION

Breast milk production occurs in the maternal breasts and relies on hormonal responses for adequate milk production.

- Formed in the acinar or alveolar cells of the mammary glands, breast milk begins to be secreted starting in the fourth month of pregnancy.
- With delivery of the placenta, progesterone levels fall dramatically, which stimulates the production of prolactin (released from the anterior pituitary gland).
- Prolactin stimulates the production of milk.
- Initiation of newborn feeding as soon as possible after birth will initiate production of prolactin-releasing factor in the hypothalamus.
- Colostrum is a thin, watery, yellow fluid that contains protein, sugar, fat, water, minerals, vitamins, and

maternal antibodies, which is produced for the first 3 to 4 days after birth.

- Transitional milk begins to form on days 2 to 4 and may be present up to 10 to 14 days after birth. It is characterized by a creamy milk, and is often referred to by mothers as "their milk coming in."
- As the baby latches on and begins to breastfeed steadily, many mothers begin to notice a tingly pins-and-needles sensation, which indicates that that the milk let-down reflex has occurred.
  - This reflex causes milk to be pushed out of the milk-producing cells into milk ducts so that it is available for feeding. The let-down reflex can be stimulated by the baby's suckling, the approach of feeding time, or just the sound of a baby crying.
- In most women, mature milk begins to appear near the end of the second week after childbirth.
- Mature milk is the final milk that is produced and is comprised of 90% water, which is necessary to maintain infant hydration. The other 10% is comprised of carbohydrates, proteins, and fats, which are necessary for both growth and energy.
  - There are two types of mature milk: foremilk and hind-milk. Ingestion of both foremilk and hind-milk is necessary to ensure the baby is receiving adequate nutrition.
    - Foremilk: This type of milk is ingested during the beginning of the feeding and contains water, vitamins, and protein.
    - Hind-milk: This type of milk is produced after the initial release of milk and contains higher levels of fat, which is necessary for weight gain.

FAST FACTS in a NUTSHELL

During the let-down reflex, the infant's suckling releases oxytocin from the posterior pituitary, which causes the collecting sinuses of the mammary glands to contract, forcing milk forward through the nipples.

Maternal Advantages of Breastfeeding

- Protective function for breast cancer
- Release of oxytocin aids in uterine involution
- Empowering effect
- Reduces cost of feeding
- Promotes optimal maternal–infant attachment

Infant Advantages of Breastfeeding

- Immunoglobulin A (IgA)—binds with large molecules of foreign proteins, including viruses and bacteria
- Lactoferrin—iron-binding protein that interferes with growth of pathogenic bacteria
- Lysozyme—destroys bacteria by dissolving cell membranes
- Bifidus factor—growth-promoting factor for lacto-bacillus bifidus, which interferes with colonization of bacteria in the gastrointestinal tract, reducing diarrhea
- Ideal electrolyte and mineral composition
- High in lactose, which easily digests sugar (rapid brain growth)
- Protein, nitrogen, and linoleic acid
- Less sodium, potassium, calcium, and phosphorus than formula
- Less potential for allergy development
- Better dental arch

Contraindications for Breastfeeding

- In the United States, mothers who are infected with HIV
- Infants who cannot digest lactose (galactose 1-phosphate uridyltransferase deficiency)
- Herpes lesions on nipples
- Mother on restricted-nutrient diet that prevents quality milk production

- Mother on medications that are inappropriate for breastfeeding
- Mother exposed to radioactive compounds
- Breast cancer

Disadvantages of Breastfeeding

- May carry microorganisms—Hepatitis B virus, cytomegalovirus, HIV, illicit and prescription drugs, tobacco, or environmental contaminants are ingested by the newborn via breast milk.

Preparation for Breastfeeding

- Because breastfeeding is both a natural and a learned process, discussion and education should begin during pregnancy.
- Breastfeeding should begin as soon after birth as possible, and the labor and delivery nurse or birth attendant should be available to assist the mother in proper latching.
- For an adequate latch it is important that the newborn open his or her mouth wide enough to grasp the nipple and areola when sucking.
- Assistance from a lactation consultant should be initiated for mothers who are struggling with early feedings.

FAST FACTS in a NUTSHELL

Milk forms in response to being used. If completely emptied, milk production will refill the breast completely; if half emptied, the breast will refill halfway, and milk production will be insufficient. New mothers need to feed every 2 to 3 hours for about 10 to 15 minutes on each breast. Bottles should not be offered until 6 weeks of age or when breastfeeding has been well established.

PROLONGED JAUNDICE IN BREASTFEEDING INFANTS

Jaundice in breastfeeding infants is caused by pregnanediol, a breakdown product of progesterone found in breast milk, which depresses action of glucuronyl transferase, the enzyme that converts indirect bilirubin to its direct form, which is excreted in bile. To avoid jaundice in their newborns, women should feed frequently in the immediate birth period because colostrum is a natural laxative that helps the newborn to pass meconium and bile. Pregnanediol remains for 24 to 48 hours.

ENGORGEMENT

Engorgement is the vascular and lymphatic congestion that arises from increased blood and lymph supply to the breast. It presents as breast distention, swelling, hardness, tenderness, and heat, and the areola may be too hard for the baby to latch onto. Prevention or treatment of engorgement includes:

- Having baby feed at more frequent intervals to empty the breast
- Applying warm packs for 20 minutes prior to feeding
- Wearing a well-fitting, supportive bra
- Standing under the shower and massaging the breast to soften it so the infant can latch on easier
- Using a breast pump after feeding to completely empty the breast
- Engorgement is a transient/temporary problem (lasts 24 hours), although some mothers may fear symptoms represent an infection.

SORE NIPPLES

Sore nipples are another common complaint of new mothers; they tend to occur during the first few days of nursing. Whether the soreness is from the strong sucking action of the infant, sucking too long after the breast is emptied, or from the improper positioning and an inappropriate release of the infant from the breast, the nurse should educate the new mother on preventive measures, including:

• Positioning the baby slightly differently for each feeding to avoid pressure on the same area of the areola.
• Changing feeding positions often (football hold, side-lying, cradle hold).
• Exposing nipples to air for 10 to 15 minutes after feeding.
• Applying vitamin E after air exposure, which may toughen nipples and prevent further irritation.
• Avoiding use of a hand pump and educating mother on manual expression.

=== *FAST FACTS in a NUTSHELL*

Breast milk kept at room temperature should be kept at 66°–72° F but should be refrigerated as soon as possible.

FORMULA FEEDING

Whether a mother develops a condition that requires her to stop breastfeeding, or it is her choice to formula feed, it is important for the nurse to support and educate the new family on proper formula preparation and feeding techniques.

Commercial Formulas

Commercial formula preparations are supervised by the Food and Drug Administration. All formulas are designed to simulate the nutritional content of breast milk and contain supplemental vitamins, most commonly iron. There are different types of formulas, including:

• Milk-based formulas, used for most full-term newborns
• Lactose-free formula, used for infants with lactose intolerance or galactosemia

- Soy formula, used for infants allergic to cow's milk protein
- Elemental formula, used for infants with protein allergies and fat malnutrition

Forms of Commercial Formulas

- Powder combined with water (lowest cost)
- Condensed liquid diluted with an equal amount of water
- Ready-to-pour
- Individually prepackaged and prepared bottles of formula (highest cost)

FAST FACTS in a NUTSHELL

Parents often change formulas in response to infant colic or fear that there is an allergic reaction to a specific brand of formula. Most colic improves spontaneously between 4 and 6 months of age. True allergies to protein, on the other hand, will persist and will present not as crying but as diarrhea, vomiting, and anemia in the newborn. In the case of a true allergy, the newborn may need to be switched to a prescribed formula.

Docosahexaenoic Acid and Arachidonic Acid

- Docosahexaenoic acid (DHA) and arachidonic acid (ARA) are fatty acids naturally passed from mother to fetus in pregnancy and are naturally occurring in breast milk.
- All infant formulas sold in the United States use the same sources of DHA and ARA.
- Different formula brands may vary in the amounts of DHA and ARA they contain.
- DHA and ARA are thought to aid in the development of the infant's brain and eyesight; their long-term benefits continue to be unknown.

DHA and ARA are fatty acids naturally found in breast milk that are important in the development of membrane constituents in the central nervous system and promote eye and brain development. Most well-conducted randomized trials show no benefit.

Calculation of Formula's Adequacy

Total fluid ingested in 24 hours must be sufficient to meet needs; 75 to 90 mL (2.5 to 3 ounces) of fluid per pound of body weight per day (150 to 200 mL/kg) are needed. Number of calories required per day is 50 to 55 calories per pound of body weight (100 to 120 kcal/kg). Add 2 or 3 ounces to infant's age in months.

Preparation for Formula

- Wash top of can with warm soapy water and rinse.
- Pour into clean bottles.
- Apply nipple; do not touch the nipple.
- Place bottle cap over nipple and refrigerate.

FAST FACTS in a NUTSHELL

Formula should never be further diluted as this will reduce its nutritional components. Mothers may intentionally water down powdered formula as a money-saving practice while not fully realizing that this negatively impacts the newborn or infant.

Effective Feeding Techniques

- Microwave will heat formula hotter in the center of the bottle than on the sides. Shake and test on wrist.
- Do not store and reuse formula.

- Obtain a comfortable position.
- Limit infants to 30-minute feedings so that calories expended overall are greater than the intake of calories.

FAST FACTS in a NUTSHELL

New parents should remember to keep the baby's head elevated and to avoid excess intake of air. The newborn should be burped after ingestion of every 10 to 15 ounces. Bottles should never be propped for feedings, as this increases the chance of suffocation.

DISCHARGE PLANNING RELATED TO INFANT FEEDING

Optimal growth for neonates and infants requires careful thought about nutrition. Interventions (or lack of them) may have long-term consequences, so discharge teaching is imperative:

- Teach about infant nutrition and answer questions parents may have related to feedings.
- Advise parents that after the first week of life newborns should have 6 to 8 wet diapers/day if achieving adequate fluid intake.
- Follow appropriate guidelines for leaving breast milk/formula out:
  - Breast Milk Rule of 5's
    - Room temperature for 5 hours
    - Refrigerate for 5 days
    - Freezer for 5 months
  - Formula Rule of 1's
    - Room temperature for 1 hour
    - Refrigerate for 1 day
    - Never freeze

Prematurity is a major cause of neonatal morbidity and mortality. Very-low-birth-weight infants are not initially fed by oral feedings and may rely on parental feedings. Oral feedings are introduced and include either breast milk or specialized premature infant formulas with added calories and nutrients. The majority of premature infants will not be discharged unless normal oral feedings can be provided by their caregiver.

Feeding Recommendations for the Premature Infant

- Premature infants require 100 to 120 kcal per kg per day to grow in order to gain a recommended 20 to 30 g (0.71 to 1.06 ounces) per day. Caloric intake should be monitored and adjusted to achieve this goal.
- Breastfeeding is the recommended feeding method.
- Breast milk fortification can be accomplished by adding fortifiers that contain additional calories, macronutrients, vitamins, calcium, and phosphorus, if needed.
- Standard formula contains 20 kcal per ounce, whereas preterm formulas provide 22 kcal per ounce and are enriched with additional protein, minerals, vitamins, and trace elements. A 24-kcal per ounce formula is generally reserved for use in the neonatal intensive care unit (NICU), but may be used in special cases when poor weight gain is diagnosed.
- Iron supplementation through the first year of life is recommended, regardless of feeding method.

Mothers of premature newborns should begin breast pumping immediately following birth and should continue pumping throughout the newborn's hospitalization. A lactation consult should be provided prior to discharge to assist the new mother with a pumping schedule, proper milk storage, and guidelines for transporting milk to the hospital for feedings while the infant remains in the NICU.

POSTNATAL GROWTH

Alterations in postnatal growth rates commonly occur in premature infants and warrant special consideration due to a reduced nutritional reserve in preterm infants. Factors associated with prematurity and low birth weight include:

- Poor postnatal growth increases the risk of neurodevelopmental impairment and poor cognitive outcomes.
- Premature growth charts are available for birth weight ranges: 1,500 g or less and 1,501 to 2,500 g (52.95 to 88.18 ounces).
- Variations in newborn growth are based on gestational age, gender, weight, genetics, and coexisting morbidities.
- "Catch-up" growth is generally considered to be achieved when the infant reaches between the 5th and 10th percentiles on a standard growth chart.
- Premature infants' catch-up growth presents first in head circumference, then in weight and length.
- After 2 years of age, a standard growth chart may be used.

5

Common Conditions Occurring in the Neonatal Period

Certain conditions occur commonly in the newborn period. Many of these adverse conditions, such as cold stress, are directly related to the newborn transition, which occurs at the time of birth. Other conditions, such as infection, may occur as a result of risk factors that occur prior to birth, at the time of birth, or in the early newborn period.

Nurses working with newborns need to have a comprehensive understanding of the pathophysiological processes that put a newborn at risk for certain commonly occurring conditions. Prompt identification of adverse conditions and proper nursing care to identify specific complications and prevent further complications are required.

During this part of the orientation, the nurse will be able to:

1. Compare and contrast the differences between newborn asphyxia and hypoxia
2. Identify proper nursing care needed to ensure a neutral thermal environment (NTE) is provided at the time of birth to prevent cold stress

3. List newborns at risk for hypoglycemia
4. Describe the different types of jaundice that affect newborns
5. Discuss the appropriate nursing care for the infant experiencing respiratory distress syndrome
6. Describe components of fluid and electrolyte balance for newborns
7. Identify possible causative agents associated with newborn infections

EQUIPMENT NEEDED

Infant warmer; blankets; hat; isolettes; k-pads; culture tubes; ventilator; bilirubin light; mask for bilirubin lights; continuous positive airway pressure (CPAP) machine; supplemental oxygen, oxygen mask, and tubing; intravenous (IV) fluids and tubing; lancet to obtain blood samples; glucometer; IV catheter; and heart-rate monitor.

ASPHYXIA

Asphyxia refers to deprivation of oxygen (hypoxia), which commonly results from a drop in maternal blood pressure or interference with blood flow to the fetal brain during delivery. This can occur as a result of inadequate circulation or perfusion, impaired respiratory effort, or inadequate ventilation after birth. Asphyxia occurs in about 4 of every 1,000 full-term births and is more common in premature births (Centers for Disease Control and Prevention [CDC], 2013b).

Possible Etiological Factors

When the placenta does not provide the fetus with enough oxygen, fetal hypoxia will result. Symptoms of low fetal oxygen states include:

- Meconium-stained amniotic fluid and umbilical cord
- Late fetal heart rate decelerations
- Bradycardia

- Prolonged labor
- Breech birth
- Placental abruption
- Maternal sedation in preterm infants

=== *FAST FACTS in a NUTSHELL*

Even though asphyxia and fetal hypoxia are not the same, fetal hypoxia is the most common cause of asphyxia.

HYPOXIA

Hypoxia, a condition in which the body is deprived of adequate oxygen, commonly occurs when the newborn fails to breathe adequately after delivery.

Potential Etiological Factors

- Prematurity
- Cord prolapse
- Cord occlusion
- Placental infarction
- Intrauterine growth restriction
- Maternal smoking

=== *FAST FACTS in a NUTSHELL*

Asphyxia, if not quickly reversed and treated, will undoubtedly lead to hypoxia and possible brain damage or death. The severity of the injury to the newborn is directly related to the severity of the asphyxia and length of time that it occurred. Cell damage occurs within minutes of the initial lack of blood flow and oxygen.

REPERFUSION INJURY

There is a second stage of damage called "reperfusion injury," which occurs after restoration of normal blood flow and reoxygenation to the brain due to the release of toxins by damaged cells. The degree of injury varies. Infants with mild or moderate asphyxia may have a full recovery, whereas infants who had prolonged oxygen deprivation may have permanent injury to the brain, heart, lungs, bowels, kidneys, or other organs.

Adverse Effects

Outcomes of newborns affected with asphyxia and hypoxia vary. Premature infants are at greatest risk to experience adverse effects, which may include:

- Heart rate variations
- Respiratory distress
- Central cyanosis
- Hypotonia
- Cerebral palsy
- Developmental disabilities
- Attention deficit hyperactivity disorder
- Impaired sight
- Complete organ failure
- Death

Nursing Considerations

Good management during labor and delivery and the early detection of nonreassuring fetal status are the best methods of preventing asphyxia. However, some cases of asphyxia cannot be predicted or prevented. In that case, asphyxia and the subsequent prevention of prolonged hypoxia require resuscitating the newborn infant. Only about 5% of newborn infants have asphyxia and require resuscitation.

Cold stress is the inability to maintain core body temperature and results in a markedly decreased body temperature (hypothermia), which results in an increase in the metabolic rate. Cold stress occurs most commonly in low-birth-weight and very-low-birth-weight (VLBW) infants. It is estimated that 27.8% of VLBW infants experience cold stress (Bissinger & Annibale, 2010).

Possible Etiological Factors

- Prematurity
- Growth-restricted infants
- Infants with asphyxia
- Infants with respiratory difficulties
- Poor environmental conditions (where heat loss is likely to occur)

Adverse Effects

Ongoing cold stress can lead to:

- Hypoglycemia
- Burning of brown fat
- Impaired weight gain
- Metabolic acidosis
- Newborn jaundice

Nursing Considerations

The best method of handling cold stress is prevention. Interventions to reduce cold stress include:

- Preventing drafts and temperature changes in the delivery room area
- Observing for signs of cold stress
- Maintaining a neutral thermal environment

- Monitoring and assessing skin temperature every 15 to 20 minutes
- Warming the baby slowly
- Increasing hourly temperature by 1° C (33.8° F) per hour until the temperature stabilizes
- Obtaining blood sugar to determine whether hypoglycemia is present
- Warming IV fluids prior to administration
- Avoiding heat loss through evaporation, convection, conduction, and radiation

Causes of Cold Stress

Glucose is necessary in larger amounts when the metabolic rate rises to produce heat; if the glycogen stores are depleted or were sparse to begin with, hypoglycemia may result. Hypoglycemia in combination with the metabolism of brown fat causes release of fatty acids, leading to acidosis. From there, the elevated fatty acids can interfere with the transport of bilirubin to the liver, leading to increased risk of jaundice. When acidosis occurs and the body attempts to conserve heat, vasoconstriction occurs and the risk of pulmonary vasoconstriction opening the patent ductus arteriosus occurs. Reverting back to fetal circulation can lead to hypoxia and can influence the left-to-right shunting, thereby increasing respiratory distress. The hazards of cold stress are included in Table 5.1.

TABLE 5.1 Hazards of Cold Stress
Increased need for oxygen
Respiratory distress
Decreased surfactant production
Hypoglycemia
Metabolic acidosis
Jaundice

Nursing Considerations

A neutral thermal environment (NTE) is the environment in which the body temperature is within the recommended range. The NTE allows for minimal oxygen and caloric consumption and the least metabolic energy expenditure. This can vary depending on the infant's age and weight. Nurses can maintain an NTE by:

- Providing external heat sources (radiant warmers, isolettes, k-pads, etc.)
- Avoiding cold exposure during procedures such as bathing and diapering
- Keeping the infant's head covered
- Swaddling the infant to conserve heat
- Keeping the infant in a flexed position to optimize warmth

HYPOGLYCEMIA

Hypoglycemia is a condition in which the amount of blood glucose in the blood is lower than normal. Blood glucose less than 40 mg/dL in the newborn period is considered normal.

The normal range of blood glucose varies depending on the age of the baby, type of food, assay method used, and possibly the mode of delivery. Up to 14% of healthy term babies may have a blood glucose level less than 40 mg/dL during the first 3 days of life.

Newborns consume fuel sources at a faster rate due to their rapid rate of breathing, loss of heat when exposed to cold, activity, and activation of muscle tone. Glucose is the main source of energy in the first 4 to 6 hours after birth and is the main source of fuel for the brain. During pregnancy, glucose is passed to the fetus from the mother through the placenta. Some of the glucose is stored as glycogen in the placenta and, later, in the fetal liver, heart, and muscles.

These stores are important for supplying the newborn's brain with glucose during delivery, and for nutrition after the baby is born. The brain depends on blood glucose as its main source of fuel, and severe or prolonged hypoglycemia may result in seizures and/or serious brain injury (Persson, 2009).

FAST FACTS in a NUTSHELL

Blood glucose should be checked on all babies who are small for gestational age or large for gestational age, have low temperatures, are jittery, or who had a stressful delivery. If the blood glucose level is below 40 mg/dL, start feeding protocol per hospital.

Possible Etiological Factors

- Inadequate maternal nutrition in pregnancy
- Cold stress
- Excess insulin production by a newborn of a diabetic mother
- Incompatibility of blood types of newborn and mother
- Birth defects and congenital metabolic diseases
- Birth asphyxia
- Liver disease

Adverse Effects

- Tremors, jitteriness, irritability
- Exaggerated Moro reflex
- High-pitched cry
- Lethargy, listlessness, hypotonia
- Cyanosis, apnea, tachypnea
- Hypothermia, temperature instability
- Poor suck, refusal to feed
- Apnea

Nursing Considerations

- Glucose screening is recommended for high-risk infants:
  - Infants whose mothers had uncontrolled gestational diabetes or diabetes mellitus
  - Large for gestational age (> 8 pounds 12 ounces or > 3,969 g)
  - Small for gestational age (< 5 pounds 12 ounces or < 2,608 g)
  - Premature (< 37 weeks gestation)
  - Low birth weight (< 2,500 g)
  - Donor twin in twin-to-twin transfusion
  - Polycythemia (hematocrit > 70%)
  - Hypothermia
  - Stress (sepsis, respiratory distress, other)
  - Low Apgar scores (< 5 at 1 minute or < 6 at 5 minutes)
- Specific treatments for hypoglycemia are based on the infant's gestational age, overall health, and medical history. Treatment options include:
  - Early feeding of rapid-acting source of glucose, such as an early feeding of a glucose/water mixture or formula.
  - During the first 4 hours of life: Any newborn glucose level less than 40 mg/dL in a baby with symptoms requires immediate IV-fluid therapy.
  - In an asymptomatic baby, with an initial glucose level of less than 25 mg/dL, an immediate feeding followed by another glucose check in an hour is indicated. If the subsequent test is still less than 25 mg/dL, immediate IV-fluid therapy is indicated.
  - Between 4 and 24 hours of life: Any glucose level less than 40 mg/dL with symptoms requires immediate IV-fluid therapy.
  - If asymptomatic and a glucose level less than 35 mg/dL, initiation of an oral feeding and another glucose check in 1 hour are indicated. If the subsequent test is still less than 35 mg/dL, immediate IV-fluid therapy is indicated (Canahuati, 1998).

FAST FACTS in a NUTSHELL

Glucose levels should be closely monitored after glucose supplementation (orally or IV) to evaluate whether the hypoglycemia occurs again.

JAUNDICE

Jaundice refers to the yellow pigmentation of the skin and conjunctival membranes caused by excess bilirubin in the blood; it occurs when the old cells break down and hemoglobin is changed into bilirubin and removed by the liver. It is estimated that over 50% of newborns will develop some amount of jaundice during the first week of life. The buildup of bilirubin in the blood is called *hyperbilirubinemia* (Wainer, 2007). The most common symptoms of jaundice include yellow coloring of the baby's skin, usually beginning on the face and moving down the body; poor feeding; or lethargy. The types of jaundice are listed in Table 5.2.

TABLE 5.2 Types of Jaundice

Physiologic jaundice: Occurs as a "normal" response to the baby's limited ability to excrete bilirubin in the first days of life; occurs after 24 hours of life; most of the time resolves without treatment.

Pathologic jaundice: Jaundice may occur with the abnormal breakdown of red blood cells due to hemolytic disease of the newborn (Rh disease), polycythemia (too many red blood cells), inadequate liver function, infection, or other factors; occurs within first 24 hours of life; needs additional medical management and may be associated with infection, metabolic disorder, bleeding disorder, liver abnormality, or a defect in excretion. Neonatal hypoxia, congenital heart disease, reduced bowel motility, and intestinal obstruction are also common causes.

Breast milk jaundice: About 2% of breastfed babies develop jaundice after the first week; monitoring is needed; should resolve without treatment.

Possible Etiological Factors

- Prematurity
- Maternal fetal incompatibility
- Cephalhematoma
- Areas of bruising
- Feeding problems
- Cold stress

═══════════════════════*FAST FACTS in a NUTSHELL*

The timing of the appearance of jaundice helps with the diagnosis. Bilirubin level peaks in a term baby at 3 to 5 days and in 5 to 7 days in a preterm baby.

═══════════════════════*FAST FACTS in a NUTSHELL*

Although low levels of bilirubin are not usually a concern, large amounts can circulate to tissues in the brain and may cause seizures and brain damage. This condition is called *kernicterus.*

Nursing Considerations

Treatment depends on many factors, including the cause of the jaundice and the level of bilirubin as well as the extent of the disease, gestational age, overall health, and medical history. The goal is to keep the level of bilirubin from increasing to dangerous levels. Key nursing interventions include:

- Identification of infants at risk
- Frequent nursing to maintain hydration and aid in excretion
- Maintaining thermoregulation
- Phototherapy
- Fiber optic blanket
- Exchange transfusion

- Increased breastfeeding
- Treatment of underlying conditions

FAST FACTS in a NUTSHELL

Maintaining the baby's temperature to decrease stress and acidosis, monitoring stools for frequency, and encouraging early breastfeeding and adequate and frequent hydration via feedings to promote intestinal colonization and calories needed for hepatic binding proteins are imperative.

RESPIRATORY DISTRESS

Transient Tachypnea of the Newborn

Transient tachypnea of the newborn (TTN; "transient" means temporary; "tachypnea" means fast breathing rate) is a term for a mild newborn respiratory problem that begins soon after birth and can last up to 3 days. Only a small percentage of all newborns develop TTN. Most babies with this problem are full term, although premature infants can also develop TTN.

Possible Etiological Factors

- Slow absorption of fluid in the fetal lungs
- Cesarean birth

Adverse Effects

- Tachypnea (over 60 breaths/minute)
- Grunting sounds with breathing
- Flaring of the nostrils
- Retractions

Nursing Considerations

Treatment for transient tachypnea of the newborn depends on gestational age, overall health, and medical history, as well as extent of the condition and the newborn's tolerance for specific medications, procedures, or therapies. Treatment options may include:

- Chest x-ray for diagnostic purposes
- Supplemental oxygen given by mask or oxygen hood
- CPAP treatment
- Mechanical ventilation
- Tube feedings

PERSISTENT PULMONARY HYPERTENSION

Persistent pulmonary hypertension (PPHN) is also known as persistent fetal circulation. The incidence of PPHN is approximately 1 in every 500 to 700 births. In this condition, a newborn circulatory system reverts back to fetal circulation due to lowered oxygen levels or difficulty breathing at birth.

Possible Etiological Factors

- Full-term or postterm pregnancies
- Traumatic birth
- Birth asphyxia

Adverse Effects

- Cyanosis
- Tachypnea
- Tachycardia
- Low blood oxygen levels, even while receiving 100% oxygen

Nursing Considerations

Treatment of PPHN is aimed at increasing oxygen to the rest of the body systems; however, long-term health problems may be related to damage from lowered oxygen in the body. Treatment for PPHN may include:

- 100% supplemental oxygen by mask or hood
- Endotracheal tube and mechanical ventilation
- Nitric oxide (to help dilate the blood vessels in the lungs)
- Extracorporeal membrane oxygenation (ECMO)—cardiopulmonary bypass during which oxygen is added and carbon dioxide is removed. ECMO is only used in specialized neonatal intensive care units (NICUs).

INFECTIONS

Newborn infants have limited ability to prevent and fight infectious diseases. Special care is needed for babies who develop an infection before, during, or after birth.

Respiratory Syncytial Virus

Respiratory syncytial virus (RSV) is a viral illness that often mimics a cold, and is the most common cause of bronchiolitis and pneumonia. It is frequently found in NICUs. Although the virus does not typically occur until 1 month of age, premature babies are at an increased risk for infection. The incubation period is 4 days. RSV is more common in the winter and spring months in the United States. Symptoms may include:

- Nasal discharge
- Apnea
- Listlessness
- Fever

- Poor feeding
- Wheezing
- Retractions
- Tachycardia
- Dry hacking cough

Possible Etiological Factors

- Spread from respiratory secretions of the eyes, mouth, or nose
- Spread through the inhalation of droplets via sneezing or coughing
- Spread through contact with contaminated objects or surfaces
- Infants with chronic lung disease are at greater risk

Adverse Effects

- Severe respiratory illness
- Pneumonia, which can become life-threatening
- Development of reactive airway disease (in later life)
- Childhood asthma

Nursing Considerations

A review of family history is important because diagnosis is aided by a history of illness in other family members, other babies in the hospital nursery, or the time of year. A swab of the baby's respiratory secretions may show the presence of a virus. Although there are no medications used to treat the virus itself, care of a baby with RSV involves treating the symptoms. Because RSV is caused by a virus, antibiotics are not useful. Interventions may include:

- Supplemental oxygen
- IV fluids
- Tube feedings
- Bronchodilator medications
- Antiviral medications (for very sick or high-risk babies)

One of the following medications, although these are not vaccines and do not prevent the virus, is usually given monthly during the RSV season (late fall through spring) to high-risk newborns to lessen the severity of the illness and help shorten the hospital stay:

- Palivizumab, an antibody against RSV
- Respiratory syncytial virus immune globulin IV (RSV-IGIV)

Group B Streptococcus

Group B streptococcus (GBS) is a bacteria that can normally be found in the digestive tract, urinary tract, and genital area of both males and females. In fact, one out of every four or five pregnant women carries GBS in her rectum or vagina. Newborns can contract GBS both during pregnancy and from the mother's genital tract during labor and delivery.

Adverse Effects

- Respiratory problems
- Changes in blood pressure
- Neurological problems, such as seizures
- Pneumonia
- Meningitis

Nursing Considerations

Possible treatment interventions for infants infected with GBS typically include:

- IV antibiotics; other treatments and specialized care may be needed
- NICU care

About 1 in every 100 to 200 babies whose mothers carry GBS develop symptoms of GBS disease. Nearly 75% of GBS cases among newborns occur in the first week of life, which is called early-onset disease. Premature babies are more susceptible to GBS infection than full-term babies (CDC, 2010; Winn, 2007).

Sepsis

Sepsis, also called sepsis neonatorum or neonatal septicemia, is a bacterial infection of the newborn. It develops from microorganisms such as bacteria, viruses, fungi, and parasites. Centers for Disease Control and Prevention statistics show that sepsis affects up to 4 in every 1,000 live births. Newborns acquire infection in one of two ways: vertical transmission, or in-utero or horizontal transmission after birth.

Possible Etiological Factors

- Premature rupture of the membranes
- Prolonged rupture of membranes (greater than 24 hours)
- Bleeding problems
- Traumatic birth
- Chorioamnionitis
- Infection of the placental tissues
- Maternal fever

Babies in the NICU are at increased risk for acquiring nosocomial (hospital-acquired) infections. Most babies in the NICU are high risk and have immature or inadequate immune systems. This makes them more susceptible to infection and more likely to need invasive treatments and procedures. Microorganisms that normally live on the skin may cause infection if they enter the body through catheters and other tubes inserted into the infant's body (Table 5.3).

TABLE 5.3 Common Microorganisms

Prenatal	During Delivery	After Birth
Rubella (German measles)	Group B streptococcus (GBS)	Respiratory syncytial virus (RSV)
Cytomegalovirus (CMV)	*E. coli*	Candida
Varicella-zoster virus	Herpes simplex virus	*Haemophilus influenzae* type B (Hib)
Listeria monocytogenes		Enterovirus

Adverse Effects

- Temperature instability (usually presents with low temperatures, rather than high)
- Respiratory problems
- Feeding intolerance
- Lethargy
- Hypoglycemia
- Apnea or difficulty breathing
- Bradycardia
- Jaundice

Nursing Considerations

A sepsis workup may be needed to help identify the location of the infection and type of microorganism causing the infection. A sepsis workup and treatment may include the following:

- Laboratory testing—blood cultures, urine samples, complete blood count, cerebrospinal fluid, C-reactive protein
- Application of broad-spectrum antibiotics
- Application of ampicillin and gentamicin
- Supportive care
  - IV fluids
  - Oxygen
  - Temperature stabilization
  - Glucose stabilization

6

High-Risk Neonatal Conditions

Multiple high-risk neonatal conditions can impact the newborn, putting the infant at risk for both short-term and long-term outcomes. The need for ongoing assessment and comprehensive care management is essential for this vulnerable population. Nurses working with high-risk newborns need to provide extensive clinical care along with education and support.

During this part of the orientation, the nurse will be able to:

1. Discuss possible adverse outcomes associated with low-birth-weight and premature newborns
2. Analyze the ongoing medical needs of newborns born to women who are HIV-positive or who have AIDS
3. Summarize care needs for newborns who are small for gestational age, who are large for gestational age, or who have intrauterine growth restriction
4. List possible adverse health outcomes associated with newborns born to diabetic mothers
5. Identify risk factors for postterm syndrome

LOW BIRTH WEIGHT

Low birth weight (LBW) is defined as a birth weight of a live-born infant less than 2,500 g (5.5 pounds), regardless of gestational age.

Very low birth weight (VLBW) is defined as a birth weight of a live-born infant less than 1,500 g (3.3 pounds).

Extremely low birth weight (ELBW) is defined as a birth weight of a live-born infant less than 1,000 g (2.2 pounds).

Possible Etiological Factors/Risk Factors

- Small parental stature/familial inheritance
- Congenital defects
- Chromosomal disorders
- Multiparity
- Previous LBW infants
- Poor nutrition
- Maternal heart disease
- Maternal hypertension
- Smoking
- Drug addiction
- Alcohol abuse
- Lead exposure
- Insufficient prenatal care

Adverse Effects

- Birth asphyxia
- Meconium aspiration
- Unstable blood sugar levels
- Developmental delays
- Psychological adjustment issues
- Intellectual disability
- Developmental delays

Nursing Considerations for the Care of the LBW Infant

- Monitor weight loss/gain in newborn period
- Frequent feedings
- Assess for respiratory problems, poor postnatal growth, and infections
- Educate parents that LBW infants are more at risk for ongoing chronic health issues
- Closely monitor achievement of developmental milestones during infancy due to increased risk of neurodevelopmental delays
- Referral for parenting interventions as appropriate

PREMATURITY

Prematurity, which occurs in 12% of births in the United States, is defined as a birth that occurs prior to 37 weeks (Davidson, London, & Ladewig, 2011). Late preterm births are those that occur between 34 and 36 weeks. Although late preterm infants typically have less significant long-term complications, the concern is that they appear "normal" but are at risk for more adverse outcomes than term infants. Very preterm infants often require extensive nursing services and are typically cared for in neonatal intensive care units (NICUs). Prematurity accounts for 75% to 80% of all neonatal morbidity and mortality (Davidson et al., 2011).

Possible Etiological/Risk Factors

- Congenital birth defects
- Preterm labor
- Low socioeconomic status
- African American race
- Maternal age less than 15 or greater than 40 years of age
- Chorioamnionitis
- Intrauterine growth restriction

- Maternal diabetes
- Multiple gestation
- Tobacco use

Adverse Effects of Prematurity

- Feeding difficulties
- Temperature intolerance
- Infections
- Prolonged jaundice
- Long-term disabilities
- Cerebral palsy
- Neurodevelopmental disabilities
- Pneumonia
- Hearing loss
- Vision deficits
- Intellectual disabilities
- Respiratory distress syndrome
- Bronchopulmonary dysplasia
- Periventricular hemorrhage/intraventricular hemorrhage
- Poorer health and social/emotional functioning measured at preschool age, in adolescence, and in young adulthood

Nursing Considerations for the Care of Infants With Prematurity

- Neonatal resuscitation team should be in attendance for delivery.
- Ensure respiratory stability immediately after birth via respiratory assessment, including pulse oximetry.
- Newborns with respiratory distress may need continuous positive airway pressure (CPAP) given nasally, by mask (Neopuff), or by using an endotracheal tube.
- Surfactant may be administered to accelerate lung maturation (recommend administration within 2 hours of birth).
- Prevent hyperoxia and hypoxia by maintaining oxygen saturation (SaO_2) between 86% and 93%.
- Perform a gestational age assessment at time of birth.

- Ensure temperature stabilization using radiant warmers, incubators, or plastic wrap with a humidified environment for ELBW newborns.
- Monitor blood sugar as needed.
- Skin care should focus on prevention of injury and preventing skin breakdown.
- Maintain adequate intravenous infusions to maintain normal fluid and electrolyte balance.
- Ensure adequate urine output for 24 hours prior to starting electrolyte replacement.
- Assess for jaundice during hospitalization and in the first few days following discharge.
- Monitor weight every 24 hours.
- Educate parents that premature infants may be behind in meeting normal developmental milestones.
- Arrange consultation with developmental pediatrician after discharge.
- Referral to early-intervention services may be warranted in infancy.
- Provide parents with accurate information and support.
- Obtain referrals for support groups or peer mentoring.
- Encourage frequent visitation, phone calls, and sibling visits after mother's discharge to facilitate attachment.
- Assist mother with breast pumping and storage of breast milk during newborn hospitalization.
- Administer car seat safety test prior to discharge.

═══════════════════════════*FAST FACTS in a NUTSHELL*

The most significant risk factor for preterm birth is a past preterm delivery.

NEWBORNS EXPOSED TO MATERNAL HIV

Perinatal transmission of HIV occurs when the fetus/newborn becomes affected with the HIV virus during pregnancy, labor, or birth, or via breastfeeding.

National Institutes of Health HIV Statistics

- In 2006, 8,700 HIV-positive women gave birth.
- Women with HIV who take antiretroviral medication during pregnancy can reduce transmission rates to less than 1%.
- Transmission risks are approximately 25% in untreated HIV-positive women.
- Transmission rates of 10% to 20% occur during labor and delivery when antiretrovirals are not administered.
- Transmission rates associated with breastfeeding are 15% at 24 months of age.
- Although the number of women with HIV giving birth is increasing, perinatal transmission rates are decreasing (National Institutes of Health [NIH], 2012).
- Perinatal transmission has decreased by 90% since the 1990s as a result of universal screening recommendations and antiretroviral medication (NIH, 2012).

Etiological/Risk Factors

- Lack of antiretroviral drug administration in pregnancy, labor, or delivery
- Premature rupture of membranes
- Invasive birth procedures
- Vaginal birth in women with high viral loads
- Instrument/operative vaginal birth

Nursing Considerations for the Care of Infants Exposed to Maternal HIV Infection

- Offer HIV testing for all infants with undocumented maternal HIV status.
- Obtain referral to social services referral.
- Obtain baseline complete blood count (CBC).
- Begin neonatal zidovudine (ZDV) therapy for first 6 weeks in newborns whose mothers received antivirals during pregnancy.

- If pharmacological intervention was initiated only during labor and not during pregnancy, the following treatment is recommended:
  - Administer neonatal dose of nevirapine at time of birth, within 48 hours of birth, and 96 hours after second dose.
  - Administer ZDV immediately at time of birth and continue for 6 weeks.
- Once infants begin pharmacological intervention, hemoglobin and neutrophil counts should be performed 4 to 6 weeks after therapy.
- If HIV status is not established until after birth, administer ZDV for 6 weeks.
- HIV-1 DNA polymerase chain reaction assay should be performed at 14 to 21 days after birth, at 1 to 2 months, and again at 4 to 6 months of age.
- HIV-1 virologic assay is the definitive test for confirmation of HIV status.
- Most infants can be diagnosed by 3 months of age.
- If HIV-1 virologic assay result is positive, immediate referral to an HIV specialist is warranted.
- *Pneumocystis* pneumonia prophylaxis is initiated after ZDV course is completed and should continue until 12 months of age.
- Assess maternal tuberculosis (TB) status and initiate screening for congenital TB.
- Compassionate parental education and support should be provided.
- Refer to a pediatric provider familiar with caring for infants of HIV-positive mothers.
- Educate to prevent opportunistic infection.
- Encourage HIV testing for family members.
- Breastfeeding is contraindicated in HIV-positive women (in the United States and developed countries).

FAST FACTS in a NUTSHELL

The most up-to-date website for HIV/AIDS management should be consulted for HIV treatment recommendations, which can be accessed at http://aidsinfo.nih.gov

INTRAUTERINE GROWTH RESTRICTION

Intrauterine growth restriction (IUGR) is an alteration in fetal growth in which the fetus's/newborn's weight is at or below the 10th percentile. Infants within the 3rd percentile were at highest risk for perinatal outcomes, including fetal/neonatal death. IUGR typically results due to alterations in placental functioning during pregnancy.

Symmetrical IUGR occurs when both head and body growth are symmetrically small, and represents 20% to 30% of all IUGR. It typically begins in the first or second trimester and is associated with poorer clinical outcomes (Davidson et al., 2011).

Asymmetrical IUGR occurs when the body is proportionally smaller than the head in growth. The majority of IUGRs (7% to 80%) involve asymmetry, which typically begins in the third trimester and is associated with better clinical outcomes (Davidson et al., 2011).

Small for gestational age (SGA) refers to an infant who is less than the 10th percentile for birth weight. *Very small for gestational age* refers to two standard deviations below the population norm or at less than the third percentile (Davidson et al., 2011).

Etiological/Risk Factors

- Preeclampsia/eclampsia
- Multiple gestation
- Placental abnormalities
- Living in high altitudes
- Congenital/chromosomal abnormalities
- Alcohol abuse
- Maternal obesity
- Clotting disorders
- Substance abuse
- Hypertension
- Heart disease
- Kidney disease
- Poor nutrition

- Smoking
- Diabetes in pregnancy, including gestational diabetes
- Anemia
- Thrombophilia

Adverse Effects Associated With IUGR

- Nonreassuring fetal status in labor
- Need for cesarean delivery
- Intraventricular hemorrhage
- Periventricular leukomalacia
- Hypoxic ischemic encephalopathy
- Necrotizing enterocolitis
- Bronchopulmonary dysplasia
- Sepsis
- Perinatal mortality

Nursing Considerations for Care of IUGR Infants

- Ensure that neonatal resuscitation team is present for delivery
- Maintain thermoregulation
- Stabilize newborn
- Monitor labs since newborn is at risk for:
  - Hypoglycemia
  - Hypocalcaemia
  - Polycythemia
  - Hyperbilirubinemia
- Screen for congenital anomalies
- Screen for congenital infection
- Specialized NICU care may be needed

LARGE FOR GESTATIONAL AGE AND INFANTS WITH MACROSOMIA

Large-for-gestational-age (LGA) newborns are defined as newborns born at or above the 90th percentile for gestational age. Approximately 9% of all births are classified as LGA, with American Indians having the highest rates (Davidson et al., 2011). *Macrosomia* refers to excessive intrauterine growth beyond a specific threshold regardless of gestational age. The incidence of macrosomia is 10% (Davidson et al., 2011). This condition is usually defined as a birth weight greater than 4,000 or 4,500 g.

Etiological Factors/Risks

- Postdate pregnancy
- Gestational diabetes
- Preexisting maternal diabetes
- Male newborn
- Genetic predisposition
- Maternal obesity
- Excessive maternal weight gain in pregnancy
- Multiparity
- Congenital anomalies
- Hydrops fetalis
- Erythroblastosis fetalis
- Use of some antibiotics (amoxicillin, pivampicillin) during pregnancy
- Genetic disorders associated with excessive fetal growth
  - Beckwith-Wiedemann syndrome
  - Sotos syndrome

Adverse Effects Associated With LGA and Macrosomia

- Birth trauma
- Shoulder dystocia
- Facial bruising
- Scalp contusions
- Brachial plexus injuries
- Operative vaginal birth
- Cesarean delivery
- Hypoglycemia
- Poor motor skills

- Feeding difficulties
- Irritability
- Difficult to arouse
- Polycythemia
- Hyperviscosity
- Hypocalcaemia
- Jaundice
- Respiratory distress
- Erb's palsy
- Increased morbidity and mortality
- Increased risks of childhood leukemia, Wilms' tumor, and osteosarcoma

Nursing Considerations for Care of LGA and Macrosomic Infants

- Have neonatal resuscitation team present at delivery
- Anticipate possible shoulder dystocia
- Anticipate possible need for cesarean birth
- Complete a gestational age assessment
- Monitor for hypoglycemia immediately following birth
- Prevent cold stress
- Obtain CBC, chemistry panel
- Assess for injuries associated with birth trauma
- Reassure parents that bruising is temporary
- When injuries are present, obtain referral for appropriate treatment and follow-up

FAST FACTS in a NUTSHELL

The most common cause of macrosomia is maternal diabetes. Infants who are born LGA are at higher risk of developing diabetes later in life.

NEWBORNS OF DIABETIC MOTHERS

Newborns of diabetic mothers may be born to women with gestational, type 1, or type 2 diabetes. Approximately 3% to 9% of infants are classified as infants of diabetic mothers. Only 8% of women who have abnormal glucose regulation during pregnancy have type 2 diabetes. Type 1 diabetes in pregnancy accounts for only 1% of all women with diabetes in pregnancy, with 92% of diabetic pregnant women having gestational diabetes (Davidson et al., 2011).

Etiological/Risk Factors

- Family history
- Native American, Black, Hispanic, and Asian race
- Maternal obesity

Adverse Effects Associated With Maternal Diabetes

- Birth injury
- Cesarean birth
- Birth defects
- Increased NICU admission rates
- Hypoglycemia
- LGA
- SGA
- Macrosomia
- Increased neonatal morbidity and mortality
- Childhood glucose intolerance
- Elevated serum insulin levels in childhood
- Childhood metabolic syndrome
- Long-term cardiovascular risks
- Neurocognitive disorders (attention deficit hyperactivity disorder, altered neurobehavioral functioning)

Nursing Considerations for Care of Infants With Diabetic Mothers

- Have neonatal resuscitation team present at delivery
- Anticipate possible shoulder dystocia

- Anticipate possible need for cesarean birth
- Evaluate respiratory status
- Provide respiratory intervention as needed
- Provide physical exam to assess for birth injury and congenital defects
- Obtain heel stick for glucose testing within 4 hours of birth
- Monitor for cold stress and temperature instability
- Provide continuous blood glucose monitoring (every 4 hours per institution protocol)
- Monitor labs for hypoglycemia, hyperbilirubinemia, and hypocalcaemia
- Provide parental education to reduce risk of childhood obesity and lifelong complications
- Encourage breastfeeding in this population

═══════════════════════*FAST FACTS in a NUTSHELL*

Approximately one third of women with gestational diabetes will develop overt diabetes within 5 years of delivery.

POSTTERM NEWBORNS

Postterm pregnancy (also known as postmature or prolonged pregnancy) refers to the birth of an infant after 42 weeks. Its incidence is 3% to 12% (Davidson et al., 2011).

Postdate pregnancy refers to the birth of an infant after the expected date of confinement has passed.

Etiological/Risk Factors

- Primiparity
- Prior postterm pregnancy
- Male fetus
- Family history
- Genetic factors

Adverse Effects

- Uteroplacental insufficiency
- Prolonged labor
- Cephalopelvic disproportion
- Shoulder dystocia
- Nonreassuring fetal status on labor
- Increased cesarean delivery
- Orthopedic injuries at birth
- Neurological injuries at birth
- Meconium and meconium aspiration
- Neonatal acidemia
- Low Apgar scores
- Macrosomia
- Hypoglycemia
- Polycythemia
- Fetal dysmaturity syndrome (postmaturity syndrome)
- Neonatal morbidity and mortality
- Stillbirth (6 times higher in postterm pregnancies)
- Sudden infant death syndrome
- Infant death in first year of life

Nursing Considerations for the Care of Postterm Newborns

- Have neonatal resuscitation team present at delivery
- Anticipate possible shoulder dystocia
- Anticipate possible need for cesarean birth
- Provide physical exam to assess for birth injury
- Obtain referral to specialist if injury occurred during birth
- Maintain thermoregulation since cold stress is common
- Assess for congenital defects
- Monitor for seizures or other signs of neurological injury
- Monitor respiratory status, since respiratory issues can occur in first 24 hours
- Monitor labs for hypoglycemia and polycythemia

7

Caring for Infants With Birth Disorders or Unexpected Outcomes

The birth of a baby typically represents a happy event, with the expectation that the new baby will be born healthy. Although some parents will know of a potential birth defect prior to the birth, others may be unaware that the newborn has any medical complications until after delivery. When a baby is born with a genetic or congenital defect, or when an unexpected birth outcome occurs, parents are often devastated and in need of intense psychosocial support and education. The nurse plays a key role in providing education about the newborn's condition, short- and long-term care needs, and referrals for immediate and long-term community-based support services for the family.

During this part of the orientation, the nurse will be able to:

1. Describe the most common types of birth disorders that occur in the newborn population
2. Identify possible etiological factors for specific birth disorders
3. Discuss possible complications that may occur as a result of specific birth disorders

4. List components of sensitive care for families with unexpected birth outcomes
5. Name nursing considerations and care measures for specific types of birth disorders or unexpected birth outcomes

GENETIC AND CONGENITAL DISORDERS

Genetic disorders (also known as genetic defects) are heritable abnormalities that are passed down from the genome or occur when new mutations occur in the DNA. "Genetic disorder" is the broad term for any defect resulting from a genetic-related etiology. The different types of genetic disorders can be inherited in a number of ways.

Congenital defects are those that are present at birth.

Chromosomal abnormalities are large-scale duplications or deletions of chromosomal segments or entire chromosomes that result in birth defects. The most common chromosomal disorder is Down syndrome, which occurs in 1 in 800 births (World Health Organization [WHO], 2013).

Mendelian disorders (single-gene disorders) occur as the result of a mutation to a single gene. It is estimated that there are over 10,000 single-gene mutation disorders. The most common is hypercholesterolemia, which has an incidence of 5% (WHO, 2013). The different modes of genetic inheritance are listed in Table 7.1.

Multifactorial inheritance disorders occur as a result of interaction between multiple genes and environments. In multifactorial disorders:

- Malformations can be mild to severe.
- In more severe cases, a greater number of genes is typically involved.
- Some disorders are more common in one gender than the other.
- If a condition occurs that is rare in that gender, an increased number of genes are likely involved.
- When a defect is present in close family members, risk of occurrence is higher.

TABLE 7.1 Different Types of Genetic Disorders

Type of Genetic Disorder	Description of Disorder	Examples of Disorders
Autosomal dominant	Only one mutated copy of the gene is necessary for a person to be affected. The affected gene overshadows the normal gene. Typically a parent is affected with the disorder. Not all newborns who inherit the gene will exhibit the disorder. Males and females are equally affected. Incidence of inheritance is 50%.	Huntington's disease Hereditary nonpolyposis colorectal cancer Neurofibromatosis type 1 and 2 Phocomelia
Autosomal recessive	Two copies of the abnormal gene must be present. An affected person usually has unaffected parents (carriers) who each carry a single copy of the mutated gene. Risk of inheritance with disease is 25%. When both parents are carriers, there is a 25% chance the child will be a carrier. Both males and females are equally affected.	Cystic fibrosis Sickle-cell disease Tay-Sachs disease Phenylketonuria Galactosemia
X-linked dominant	Caused by mutations in genes on the X chromosome. Although it is extremely rare, females and males can inherit, but males are more severely affected. When the father is the carrier, male offspring are not affected; however, the female offspring would be. (There is no male-to-male inheritance.) When the woman is the carrier, 50% of offspring are affected.	X-linked hypophosphatemic rickets Rett's syndrome Klinefelter syndrome

(continued)

TABLE 7.1 Different Types of Genetic Disorders (continued)

Type of Genetic Disorder	Description of Disorder	Examples of Disorders
X-linked recessive	Mutations in genes on the X chromosome that are manifested by the male who is the carrier of the abnormal gene through the female line. Men are more commonly affected. Carrier mothers will have 50% of male offspring affected, and 50% of female offspring will become carriers. Fathers cannot pass on the disorder to male offspring, but all female offspring will become carriers.	Hemophilia A Duchenne muscular dystrophy Lesch-Nyhan syndrome Male pattern baldness Red–green color blindness Turner's syndrome Fragile X syndrome
Y-linked	Only males are affected. Mutations occur from affected fathers. Female offspring are not affected. Very rare.	Azoospermia Oligospermia Gonadal dysgenesis
Mitochondrial DNA	Also known as maternal inheritance. Only mothers can pass these disorders on to their offspring.	Leber's hereditary optic neuropathy

CARING FOR INFANTS WITH BIRTH DISORDERS OR UNEXPECTED OUTCOMES

- When multiple family members have the same defect, risk increases.
- Once a specific defect occurs in one pregnancy, risk of reoccurrence is higher in subsequent pregnancies.

Nursing Considerations for Newborns With Genetic Disorders

When an infant is born with a suspected genetic disorder, nursing care should include the following:

- Obtain a detailed comprehensive family history.
- Relay information to parents in terms they can understand, including suspected diagnosis.
- Encourage parents to ask questions and express feelings.
- Draw a karyotype to confirm diagnosis.
- Perform a complete physical examination with laboratory testing, ultrasound screening, or other diagnostic testing to determine underlying complications.
- Obtain referral to appropriate support groups, peer mentoring, or support networks.
- Obtain referral to specific medical specialists for newborn evaluation.
- Consult with genetic specialist or genetics counselor as soon as possible after birth.
- Obtain referral for psychological support, counseling, grief counseling, or pastoral care.

═══════════════════════*FAST FACTS in a NUTSHELL*

Parents may feel disbelief, anger, confusion, incredible sadness, blame, jealousy, heartache, emptiness, shame, a sense of unfairness, guilt, and intense grief when their newborn is diagnosed with a genetic disorder.

CONGENITAL CARDIAC DEFECTS

Congenital cardiac defects are abnormalities in the heart's structure that occur as a result of incomplete or abnormal development in utero or as a result of a genetic defect. The incidence of congenital cardiac defects is 8 in 1,000 births. Clinical outcomes can be mild to severe in nature. Table 7.2 lists common cardiac defects.

CRITICAL CONGENITAL HEART DEFECTS

Critical congenital heart defects (CCHDs) account for 30% of infant deaths related to birth defects. Infants with CCHDs often need extensive medical intervention and usually need surgical intervention within the first 12 months of life. All infants should be screened with bedside pulse oximetry 24 to 48 hours after birth (as late as possible) to check for possible CCHDs. CCHDs include:

- Coarctation of the aorta
- Double-outlet right ventricle
- D-transposition of the great arteries
- Ebstein anomaly
- Hypoplastic left heart syndrome
- Interrupted aortic arch
- Pulmonary atresia (intact septum)
- Single ventricle
- Total anomalous pulmonary venous connection
- Tetralogy of Fallot
- Tricuspid atresia
- Truncus arteriosus

Nursing Considerations for the Care of Newborns With Cardiac Defects

- Complete physical with monitoring of heart rate and blood pressure and documentation of any cyanosis
- Bedside pulse oximetry to determine whether critical congenital heart defect is present

TABLE 7.2 Common Cardiac Defects

Type of Defect	Incidence	Description of Defect	Clinical Treatment and Anticipated Outcome
Aortic stenosis	Occurs in 5 out of every 10,000 live births. Accounts for 5% of all congenital heart disease (Congenital and Children's Heart Center, 2013).	Aortic valve is stiffened with stenosis present. Due to the narrowing and improper opening, the left ventricle works harder and is strained.	Mild cases are usually followed and do not require intervention but may warrant treatment later in life. Severe cases may require balloon dilation valvuloplasty performed via the umbilical artery. In very severe cases or when defects related to the size of the ventricles is a concern, the Ross procedure, an aortic valve replacement procedure, may be considered. The Konno procedure is sometimes considered for severe cases with severe malformations, or a Ross–Konno combination procedure may be performed for these cases. Prognosis is good, with children leading normal lives. A second surgery is sometimes needed later in life.
Atrial septal defect	Occurs in 8 out of 10,000 births. Accounts for 8% of congenital heart disease (Congenital and Children's Heart Center, 2013).	Septum between the left atrium and the right atrium occurs, which allows extra blood flow from the left atrium into the right heart and out to the lungs.	Small holes often close in the first few years of life. Larger septums require surgical intervention. Often closure during a cardiac cauterization is performed. Open surgical repairs are rarely needed. Prognosis is excellent.

(continued)

TABLE 7.2 Common Cardiac Defects (continued)

Type of Defect	Incidence	Description of Defect	Clinical Treatment and Anticipated Outcome
Atrioventricular canal defect (ACD) (endocardial cushion defect; atrioventricular septal defect)	Accounts for 5% of all congenital heart disease. Present in 15%–20% of newborns with Down syndrome.	Poorly formed central area of the heart with a large hole between the atria and ventricles. Instead of two separate valves allowing flow into the heart, there is often one large common valve, which is often malformed, that is present instead of the tricuspid on the right and mitral valve on the left.	Common in Down syndrome. Diuretics and angiotensin-converting enzyme (ACE) inhibitors are used, but all require surgical repair. Closures for the holes or patches are placed. Infants with complete ACD have surgery at 3–6 months and those with partial ACD can wait until 12–28 months. Survival rate is 96% and reoperation rate is 11%, with 10-year survival rates of 81%–91% (Pettersen & Niash, 2013).
Coarctation of the aorta	Occurs in 5 out of 10,000 births. Accounts for 6% of congenital heart disease (Congenital and Children's Heart Center, 2013).	Narrowing of a portion of the aorta seriously decreases systemic blood flow.	Prostaglandins often given in newborn period to stimulate heart. Balloon angioplasty with stent placement may be warranted. Good prognosis with no adverse effects is typical, although a repeat surgical procedure is sometimes needed later in life.

(continued)

TABLE 7.2 Common Cardiac Defects (continued)

Type of Defect	Incidence	Description of Defect	Clinical Treatment and Anticipated Outcome
Hypoplastic left heart syndrome	Occurs in 1 out of every 4,344 births (Centers for Disease Control and Prevention [CDC], 2013c).	Structures of the left side of the heart (the left ventricle, the mitral valve, and the aortic valve) are underdeveloped and poor systemic circulation occurs.	Diuretics may be administered. Feeding tubes may be needed. Surgical intervention begins at 2 weeks of age with the Norwood procedure, in which a "new" aorta is constructed and connected to the right ventricle. A bidirectional Glenn shunt procedure is performed at 4–6 months to connect the pulmonary artery to the superior vena cava. Finally, a Fontan procedure is performed at 18 months–3 years of age to attach the pulmonary artery to the inferior vena cava. Lifelong complications are common and a heart transplant is sometimes needed (CDC, 2013c).
Patent ductus arteriosus (PDA)	Occurs in 6 out of 10,000 births. Accounts for 7% of congenital heart disease (Congenital and Children's Heart Center, 2013).	Failure of the ductus arteriosus to close after birth, which results in excessive blood flow to the lungs.	Common in premature newborns. In preterm infants, indomethacin or ibuprofen may be given during first 2 weeks of life to facilitate closure. Surgical closure during first year if large hole persists. Cardiac cauterization may be used after first year if PDA persists and causes symptoms. Excellent prognosis with normal exercise tolerance expected.

(continued)

TABLE 7.2 Common Cardiac Defects (continued)

Type of Defect	Incidence	Description of Defect	Clinical Treatment and Anticipated Outcome
Pulmonary atresia	Occurs in 7.1–8.1 per 100,000 live births. Accounts for 0.7%–3.1% of patients with congenital heart disease (CDC, 2013c).	Either absence of pulmonary valve or pulmonic valve does not open. The main blood vessel that runs between the right ventricle and the lungs might also be malformed, and the right ventricle can be abnormally small in size.	Cyanosis occurs and immediate intervention needed. Systemic-to-pulmonary artery shunt placement is performed. Survival rates are 65%–82% at age 1 year and 64%–76% at age 5 years (CDC, 2013c).
Pulmonary stenosis	Occurs in 8 in 10,000 births. Accounts for 8% of congenital heart disease (Congenital and Children's Heart Center, 2013).	Pulmonic valve is stiffened and stenotic or does not open properly. Potential strain on the right side of the heart because the right ventricle has to pump harder to oxygenate lungs.	If mild, pulmonary stenosis may never require any treatment; prostaglandins may be given for severe narrowing. Surgical intervention via cardiac cauterization is rarely needed. Excellent prognosis. Follow-up surgical intervention sometimes needed later in life.

(continued)

TABLE 7.2 Common Cardiac Defects (continued)

Type of Defect	Incidence	Description of Defect	Clinical Treatment and Anticipated Outcome
Tetralogy of Fallot	Occurs 5 in 10,000 births. Accounts for 5% of congenital heart disease (Congenital and Children's Heart Center, 2013).	Four defects, including a pulmonary stenosis, ventricular hypertrophy, ventricular septal defect, and an aorta that can receive blood from both the left and right ventricles, instead of draining just to the left side.	More common in DiGeorge syndrome. Familial inheritance patterns. If symptomatic, beta-blockers can be administered in newborn period. A modified Blalock–Taussig shunt may be placed. Open surgical repair at 6–12 months is common with cardiopulmonary bypass. Prognosis is excellent but some exercise intolerance may occur. Follow-up surgery sometimes needed.
Total anomalous pulmonary venous connection	Occurs in 0.6–1.2 in 10,000 births (CDC, 2013c). Accounts for 0.7%–1.5% of congenital heart disease (CDC, 2013c).	Defect in the pulmonary veins in which the veins do not lead to the left atrium but instead deliver blood to the heart by other narrowed pathways. Increased pressure pushes fluid into the lungs, decreasing oxygenated blood that reaches the body. Three different types: supracardiac, cardiac, and infracardiac.	Respiratory distress and cyanosis may be present at birth. Prostaglandins are administered initially. If a complete obstruction is present, surgical intervention is immediate; otherwise, surgery is typically performed within 1 month. Prognosis is very good, although some exercise intolerance may occur.

(continued)

TABLE 7.2 Common Cardiac Defects (*continued*)

Type of Defect	Incidence	Description of Defect	Clinical Treatment and Anticipated Outcome
Transposition of the great arteries	Occurs in 4 in 10,000 births. Accounts for 4% of congenital heart disease (Congenital and Children's Heart Center, 2013).	Reversal of blood vessels in which the pulmonary artery and the aorta are switched so that the aorta arises from the right side of the heart and receives unoxygenated blood, which then circulates through the body. The pulmonary artery arises from the left side of the heart, receives oxygenated blood, and sends it back to the lungs again.	Severe cyanosis can occur. Prostaglandin administration necessary during newborn period. Balloon atrial septostomy is performed via the umbilical artery. A "switch procedure" is later performed to place the arteries in the correct position. Prognosis is excellent.
Tricuspid atresia	Occurs in 1 in 10,000 births. Accounts for 0.3%–3.7% of patients with congenital heart disease (CDC, 2013c).	The tricuspid valve is replaced by a nonopening plate or membrane so the right ventricle does not receive blood normally and is often congenitally small.	Shunt procedures are typically performed during the first year of life. Digitalis and diuretics may be used if congestive heart failure occurs. If palliative care measures alone are used, there is a 50% fatality rate.

(continued)

TABLE 7.2 Common Cardiac Defects *(continued)*

Type of Defect	Incidence	Description of Defect	Clinical Treatment and Anticipated Outcome
Truncus arteriosus	0.72 in 10,000 births. Approximately 300 cases in the United States annually (CDC, 2013c).	The formation of two separate vessels fails to occur, and instead a single common great blood vessel called the truncus arteriosus is present. A hole between the ventricles is also common. The valve leading into the truncus arteriosus may be very abnormal.	Digitalis, diuretics, and prostaglandins are commonly administered until a surgical repair can be performed. Complete primary repair is required to fix defects. Postoperative mortality is 10%. Survival at 10–20 years is 80%.
Ventricular septal defect	Occurs in 3 in 1,000 births. Accounts for one third of cases of congenital heart disease (Congenital and Children's Heart Center, 2013).	A septum between the heart's left and right ventricles.	Most common congenital cardiac defect. Mild cases require no intervention. Diuretics and sometimes ACE inhibitors can be used for treatment. Large defects may require a surgical repair. Multiple small holes may require a staged repair. Excellent prognosis. Close observation is warranted because irreversible lung damage can occur if not properly managed, but is rare.

- Assess for any family history of congenital cardiac disorders/disease.
- Electrocardiogram
- Echocardiogram
- Possible chest x-ray
- Possible cardiac catheterization
- Provide factual information and updates on newborn's condition.
- Referral/consultation with pediatric cardiologist
- Life-threatening cardiac defects may warrant transfer to a higher level acute care facility for intensive care services or immediate surgical intervention.
- Provide emotional support and referrals for community-based support groups/resources.
- If infant is transferred, provide detailed referral of hospital information for parents.
- Determine whether early maternal discharge can be facilitated.

CLEFT LIP AND PALATE DEFECTS (OROFACIAL CLEFTS)

Orofacial clefts occur as an isolated defect in 70% of cases, meaning there are no other associated defects present. The incidence of cleft palate is 1 in 2,651, whereas the incidence of cleft lip with or without an associated palate is 1 in 4,437 (CDC, 2013b). Orofacial defects can be caused from environmental factors, genetic abnormalities, medication exposure, or nutritional deficits.

Cleft Lip Defects

- Defects occur between the fourth and seventh gestational weeks during pregnancy.
- Occur when the tissue fails to form over the lip
- Can be a small slit or large opening
- Often unilateral but can occur in the middle of the lip (rare)

Cleft Palate Defects

- Defects occur between sixth and ninth gestational weeks during pregnancy.
- Occur when the tissue that makes up the roof of the mouth does not join correctly
- Can include the front and back portion or a small section of the palate

Complications Related to Cleft Lip and Cleft Palate

- Feeding difficulties
- Speech delays/alterations
- Dental problems
- Ear infections
- Hearing loss

Nursing Considerations for the Care of Newborns With Cleft Lip and Cleft Palate

- Assess for presence of other birth defects.
- Parents need factual information about the defects.
- Parents need emotional support and opportunities to grieve.
- Consultation with surgeon about plan of care should be scheduled early.
- Because breathing, hearing, speech, and language can be affected, referrals to appropriate specialists are warranted.
- Feeding consult is warranted for feeding issues.
- Breastfeeding may not be possible.
- Specialized bottles should be provided to aid in feeding.
- Close observation for adequate fluid intake and weight gain are important as feeding difficulties are common.
- Hearing screening is especially important in this population.
- Prompt surgery may be warranted if breathing or other severe complications are present.
- Surgical intervention is warranted by 12 months for infants with cleft lip and 18 months for infants with cleft palate.

INBORN ERRORS OF METABOLISM

Individual inborn errors of metabolism (IEMs) are relatively rare, although they are life-threatening, and result from single-gene defects. IEM disorders can involve either toxic accumulation or may be related to energy production/utilization disorders. Individual IEMs are rare, although collectively, they occur in 1 in 4,000 births. The most common inborn errors of metabolism are listed in Table 7.3.

Toxic Accumulation Defects

- Disorders of protein metabolism (amino acidopathies, organic acidopathies, urea cycle defects)
- Disorders of carbohydrate intolerance
- Lysosomal storage disorders

Energy Production and Utilization Defects

- Fatty acid oxidation defects
- Disorders of carbohydrate utilization or production (glycogen storage disorders, disorders of gluconeogenesis and glycogenolysis)
- Mitochondrial disorders
- Peroxisomal disorders

Adverse Effects and Complications

- Acute sepsis with no risk factors (occurs in 20% of affected newborns)
- Temperature instability
- Rapid deterioration after initial normal newborn course
- Neurological changes
  - Severe onset of ataxia
  - Seizures
  - Irregular movements
  - Posturing
  - Abnormal tone
  - Altered /changes in level of consciousness
- Hepatoencephalopathy

TABLE 7.3 Inborn Errors of Metabolism

Type of IEM	Incidence	Clinical Symptomology	Inheritance Pattern
Phenylketonuria	1:15,000	Intellectual disability, microcephaly	Autosomal recessive
Maple syrup urine disease	1:150,000	Acute encephalopathy, metabolic acidosis, intellectual disability	Autosomal recessive
Galactosemia	1:40,000	Hepatocellular dysfunction, cataracts	Autosomal recessive
Glycogen storage disease, type Ia (von Gierke's disease)	1:100,000	Hypoglycemia, lactic acidosis, ketosis	Autosomal recessive
Medium-chain acyl-CoA dehydrogenase deficiency	1:15,000	Nonketotic hypoglycemia, acute encephalopathy, coma, sudden infant death syndrome	Autosomal recessive
Pyruvate dehydrogenase deficiency	1:200,000	Hypotonia, psychomotor retardation, failure to thrive, seizures, lactic acidosis	X-linked
Gaucher's disease	1:60,000 (increased to 1:1,900 in Ashkenazi Jews)	Coarse facial features, hepatosplenomegaly	Autosomal recessive

(continued)

TABLE 7.3 Inborn Errors of Metabolism (continued)

Type of IEM	Incidence	Clinical Symptomology	Inheritance Pattern
Fabry's disease	1:80,000–1:117,000	Acroparesthesias, angiokeratomas, hypohidrosis, corneal opacities, renal insufficiency	X-linked
Hurler's syndrome	1:100,000	Coarse facial features, hepatosplenomegaly	Autosomal recessive
Methylmalonica ciduria	1:20,000	Acute encephalopathy, metabolic acidosis, hyperammonemia	Autosomal recessive
Propionic aciduria	1:50,000	Metabolic acidosis, hyperammonemia	Autosomal recessive
Zellweger syndrome	1:50,000	Hypotonia, seizures, liver dysfunction	Autosomal recessive
Ornithine transcarbamylase deficiency	1:70,000	Acute encephalopathy	X-linked

- Organomegaly
- Poor perfusion
- Tachypnea
- Bradycardia
- Apnea
- Acute organ dysfunction
- Multisystem organ failure
- Feeding/gastrointestinal changes
  - Poor feeding
  - Vomiting
  - Failure to thrive
  - Lethargy
- Developmental delays
- Failure to reach developmental milestones/loss of milestones
- Skeletal deformities
  - Dysmorphic features
  - Skeletal abnormalities
- Cardiopulmonary compromise
- Coma
- Unexplained newborn/infant death

Nursing Considerations for the Care of Newborns With Inborn Errors of Metabolism

- Obtain extensive family history (including family history of unexplained newborn/infant death).
- Ensure tandem mass spectrometry testing is performed as late as possible prior to discharge.
- Initial physical exam may be normal, but alterations can begin occurring as early as 24 hours after birth, with rapid deterioration common.
- Immediate transfer to a tertiary care facility is essential.
- If IEMs are suspected, comprehensive laboratory testing includes complete blood count; serum electrolytes; bicarbonate; blood gases; blood urea nitrogen; creatinine levels; bilirubin level; transaminase levels; prothrombin time; activated partial thromboplastin time; blood glucose; lactate dehydrogenase; aldolase; creatinine kinase;

and urinary testing, including pH, ketones, and urine myoglobin levels.
- Imaging studies may include electrocardiogram, radiography, computed tomography, magnetic resonance imaging, ultrasonography, and/or echocardiogram.
- Obtain enzyme assay or DNA analysis.
- If laboratory findings are abnormal, prompt consultation with an IEM specialist is warranted.
- Obtain guidelines and algorithms from the American College of Medical Genetics.
- If newborn death occurs, diagnostic testing should be performed to determine risk factors for future pregnancies and screening for siblings who could be asymptomatic.
- Emergency treatment includes immediate NPO (nothing orally) status, intravenous D10 to stabilize blood sugar levels, correction of metabolic acidosis if present, elimination of toxic metabolites, and administration of cofactors specific for the treatment of IEM.
- Some IEMs will require specific replacement enzymes.
- Specialized formulas are required and individualized based on specific type of IEM.
- Referrals for psychological counseling and community-based support are warranted.
- Organ transplants, enzyme therapy, and gene therapy required as needed
- Extensive parent education is imperative.
- Lifelong management required
- Dietary strategies typically include protein restriction and avoidance of fasting.
- Stressors, including dietary changes, trauma, or surgery, can worsen symptoms.

FAST FACTS in a NUTSHELL

Every state is required by law to screen for at least 29 IEMs. Some states screen for over 50 IEMs. Screening thresholds are intentionally set low to avoid false negatives, so false positives can occur.

Hematological disorders encountered in the newborn period include inherited clotting deficiencies (factor VIII deficiency) or acquired disorders such as hemorrhagic disease of the newborn, thrombocytopenia, newborn anemia, disseminated intravascular coagulation (DIC), and liver failure.

Hemorrhagic Disease of the Newborn

Hemorrhagic disease in the newborn infant is caused by the deficiency of the vitamin K-dependent clotting factors (II, VII, IX, and X) and occurs in 0.25% to 1.7% of newborns who have not received vitamin K administration after birth. In newborns with hemorrhagic disease:

- Vitamin K was typically not given after birth.
- Bleeding occurs within 5 days to 6 weeks.
- Bleeding sites may include the gastrointestinal tract, umbilical cord, circumcision site, and nose.
- Risk for intracranial hemorrhage
- Increased risk in infants of mothers taking hydantoin anticonvulsants or warfarin
- Increased incidence in breastfed infants
- DIC and hepatic failure must be ruled out.
- Intravenous vitamin K is administered; injections are contraindicated.

Thrombocytopenia

Thrombocytopenia is defined as a platelet count under 150,000/μL (usually less than 50,000/μL, may be less than 10,000/μL). It can be idiopathic or related to deficiency of clotting factors. Newborns affected by Rh isoimmunization are at risk for isoimmune thrombocytopenia.

In newborns with thrombocytopenia:

- Transfusion is necessary for term newborn if total platelet count is less than 20,000/μL or active bleeding is present.
- Transfusion is necessary for preterm infant if there is a risk for intraventricular hemorrhage or if the total platelet count is less than 40,000/μL.
- Isoimmune thrombocytopenia requires transfusions with maternal platelets until platelet counts reach 50,000/μL or higher.
- Newborns born to mothers with idiopathic thrombocytopenic purpura do not typically need treatment; if bleeding occurs, prednisone 2 mg/kg/day is given for 7 to 14 days.

Newborn Anemia

Anemia can occur as a result of hemorrhage, hemolysis, or failure to produce red blood cells. Newborn hemorrhage can occur as a result of:

- In utero etiologies (fetoplacental and fetomaternal)
- Perinatal etiologies (cord rupture, placenta previa, placenta abruption)
- After birth (intracranial hemorrhage, cephalohematoma, ruptured liver or spleen)

Hemolysis, which is almost always associated with hyperbilirubinemia, can occur as a result of multiple etiologies, including:

- Blood group incompatibilities
- Enzyme abnormalities
- Membrane abnormalities
- Infection
- DIC

Polycythemia

Polycythemia is categorized by a capillary hematocrit that is greater than 68% or a venous hematocrit greater than 65%. In newborns with polycythemia, hyperviscosity with decreased perfusion of the capillary beds occurs. Polycythemia occurs in 2% to 5% of all live births and occurs more commonly in newborns who are small for gestational age or large for gestational age. Common etiologies include:

- Twin–twin transfusion
- Maternal–fetal transfusion
- Intrapartum transfusion from the placenta
- Chronic intrauterine hypoxia

Treatment is warranted for all symptomatic infants. Treatment for symptomatic newborns varies. The recommended treatment includes:

- Isovolumic partial exchange transfusion with 5% albumin or normal saline
- Blood is withdrawn from the umbilical artery while the infusion is administered over 15 to 30 minutes
- Obtaining a desired hematocrit value of 50% to 55%
- Obtaining a blood volume of 80 mL/kg

Inherited Hemolytic Anemias

Inherited hemolytic anemias are associated with genetic defects that control red blood cell production (Table 7.4).

Disseminated Intravascular Coagulation

DIC is a condition of uncontrolled bleeding that occurs with simultaneous uncontrolled clotting, which occurs when inappropriate activation and consumption of clotting

TABLE 7.4 Types of Inherited Hemolytic Anemias

Type of Inherited Anemia	Abnormality	Population Affected
Sickle cell anemia	Abnormally shaped hemoglobin, which are sickle- or crescent-shaped and have decreased oxygen-carrying capabilities. Red blood cells have a shorter life span. Bone marrow cannot make enough red blood cells to meet needs.	African Americans
Thalassemia	Decreased hemoglobin levels. This causes the body to make fewer healthy red blood cells than normal.	People of Southeast Asian, Indian, Chinese, Filipino, Mediterranean, or African origin or descent
Hereditary spherocytosis	Defect in the surface membrane of red blood cells causes them to have a sphere, or ball-like, shape. These blood cells have a life span that is shorter than normal.	Northern European descent
Hereditary elliptocytosis (ovalocytosis)	Cell membrane abnormality in which the red blood cells are elliptic (oval) in shape. They are not as flexible as normal red blood cells, and they have a shorter life span.	
Glucose-6-phosphate dehydrogenase (G6PD) deficiency	Lack of G6PD enzyme results in red blood cells rupturing when they come into contact with certain substances in the bloodstream.	Males of African or Mediterranean descent; African American males
Pyruvate kinase deficiency	Lack of pyruvate kinase causes early cell death and breakdown.	Amish

factors result in a hemorrhagic state because of inadequate hemostasis. The most common etiologies include:

- Asphyxia
- Hypoxemia
- Shock
- Acidosis
- Sepsis
- Respiratory distress syndrome
- Hyaline membrane disease

Adverse Effects and Consequences of DIC

- Uncontrolled bleeding
  - Petechiae
  - Purpura
  - Ecchymoses
  - Hematomas
- Ischemic damage
- Organ failure
- Death

Treatment Strategies for DIC

- Monitor laboratory values for progression of disorder
- Identify and correct underlying cause
- Administer a antibiotics if infection present
- Administer transfusions of platelets and/or fresh frozen plasma
- Administer transfusions of packed red blood cells to correct anemia
- Provide ventilator assistance
- Administer vasopresser drips
- Monitor vital signs
- Monitor fluid and electrolyte balance
- Provide nutritional support
- Avoid venipuncture and invasive procedures

Nursing Considerations for Newborns With Hematological Disorders

- Obtain pregnancy, labor, and birth history.
- Obtain family history of genetic hematological disorders.
- Obtain parental ethnic group to determine risk factors for inherited disorders.
- Provide laboratory testing to determine type of hematological disorder.
- Provide immediate treatment to correct disorder.
- Administer medications or blood products.

8

Special Topics
for Neonatal Care

The care of newborns and their families often involves complex issues. Some infants are born after exposure to substances, alcohol, and tobacco, putting them at an increased risk for both immediate and long-term adverse health outcomes. Other infants are born on the edge of viability and will require initial decision making on the appropriate care to be given at the time of birth. Some of these neonates may be provided with palliative care measures, whereas others may receive resuscitation measures. These cases usually involve complex decision making laced with ethical, legal, and emotional implications. These infants, along with other critically ill infants, often warrant interventions that will involve neonatal surgery. The neonate represents multiple challenges when undergoing surgical intervention, including the use of anesthesia when the newborn is not stable. Many of these newborns will need to be transferred to facilities that can meet their unique care needs.

During this part of the orientation, the nurse will be able to:

1. Identify possible newborn complications associated with substance abuse, alcohol, and tobacco exposure
2. Describe the ethical issues involved in decision making for an infant born on the edge of viability
3. List the most common surgical procedures performed in the newborn period
4. Discuss the complication that may occur in newborns receiving anesthesia
5. Delineate the essential skills required for neonatal transport team members to ensure safe transfer for critically ill newborns

NEWBORNS EXPOSED TO SUBSTANCE ABUSE, ALCOHOL, AND TOBACCO

Substance abuse in pregnancy can create adverse maternal, fetal, and neonatal outcomes. A comprehensive review is needed to determine whether there is any history of a substance abuse problem/disorder and, whether so, the mother's previous drug-use patterns. Prenatal, labor, and birth history should also be obtained. It is important to illicit information in a nonthreatening, nonjudgmental way.

ALCOHOL USE IN PREGNANCY

Alcohol use continues in 7.6% of pregnant women, with 12.2% of pregnant women consuming at least one alcohol-containing beverage within the last 30 days. Of those women who continually use alcohol during pregnancy, 1.4% are classified as binge drinkers (drinking more than six drinks on one occasion). Of women who binge drink in pregnancy, the average frequency of episodes was three times per month (Centers for Disease Control and Prevention [CDC], 2012). Characteristics of women who use alcohol in pregnancy include (CDC, 2012):

- Aged 35 to 44 years (14.3%)
- White (8.3%)

- College graduate (10.0%)
- Unmarried (13.4%)
- Employed (9.6%)

═══════════════════════════*FAST FACTS in a NUTSHELL*

The strongest predictor for alcohol use in pregnancy is past use prior to conception. A detailed history on alcohol use patterns prior to pregnancy is important to determine the risk of use and continuation during the prenatal period.

FETAL ALCOHOL SPECTRUM DISORDERS

Fetal alcohol spectrum disorders (FASDs) are a group of conditions that can occur in a person who is exposed to alcohol in utero. The effects of alcohol consumption may include physical alterations and behavioral or learning disorders.

Types of FASDs

Fetal Alcohol Syndrome

Fetal alcohol syndrome (FAS) is the most severe disorder on the FASD spectrum and often results in fetal death. FAS is associated with a combination of the following:

- Abnormal facial features
- Growth problems
- Central nervous system issues
- Learning, memory, attention span, and communication deficits
- Vision problems
- Hearing loss
- Difficulty interacting with others

Alcohol-Related Neurodevelopmental Disorder

Alcohol-related neurodevelopmental disorder commonly results in a variety of impairments, including:

- Intellectual disabilities
- Behavioral problems
- Learning disabilities
- Poor school performance with:
  - Math
  - Memory
  - Attention
  - Judgment
  - Poor impulse control

Alcohol-Related Birth Defects

People with alcohol-related birth defects have birth defects that include:

- Vision or hearing problems
- Cardiac defects
- Impairment of kidneys
- Skeletal disorders

SUBSTANCE ABUSE IN PREGNANCY

Approximately 4% of pregnant women are drug dependent during pregnancy. Commonly used substances include marijuana, cocaine, ecstasy and other amphetamines, and heroin. Substance abuse in pregnancy has been associated with adverse fetal and newborn outcomes. Tobacco use in pregnancy continues in 10.4% of pregnancies. The adverse effects vary depending on the type of substance used.

Marijuana is associated with:

- Premature birth
- Small for gestational age
- Withdrawal symptoms after birth
- Difficulty with state regulation after birth
- Poor sleep patterns

- Increased sensitivity to environmental stimuli
- Learning disabilities
- Behavioral problems

Ecstasy, methamphetamine, and other amphetamines are associated with:

- Small for gestational age
- Intrauterine growth restriction
- Congenital heart defects
- Club foot (found only in female fetuses)
- Small head circumference
- Placental disorders
- Cleft lip/cleft palate
- Learning disabilities
- Behavioral problems

Heroin use in pregnancy is associated with:

- Intrauterine growth restriction
- Low birth weight
- Premature rupture of the membranes
- Premature birth
- Withdrawal symptoms after birth
- Learning disabilities
- Behavioral problems
- Physical disabilities
- Stillbirth
- Sudden infant death syndrome (SIDS)

Cocaine use in pregnancy is associated with:

- Premature birth
- Low birth weight
- Intrauterine growth restriction
- Cerebral palsy
- Placenta abruption
- Behavioral difficulties
- Urinary tract defects
- Language delays
- Alterations in growth until the age of 10

Club drug use (phenylcyclidine [PCP/angel dust], ketamine [Special K], and lysergic acid diethylamide [LSD/acid]) in pregnancy is associated with:

- Neonatal withdrawal
- Behavioral problems
- Learning disabilities

Glue and solvent use in pregnancy is associated with:

- Intrauterine growth restriction
- Preterm birth
- Fetal loss
- Birth defects

Tobacco use in pregnancy is associated with:

- Small for gestational age
- Preterm birth
- Placental disorders
- Low birth weight
- SIDS
- Cleft lip/cleft palate

NEONATAL ABSTINENCE SYNDROME

Neonatal abstinence syndrome (NAS) describes a group of problems that occur in newborns who have been exposed to addictive illegal or prescription drugs in utero. Babies of mothers who consume alcohol during pregnancy may have a similar condition. These infants continue to have risks for adverse health outcomes that continue in the neonatal period and during the first year of life, with some having life-long adverse health conditions and implications. Due to the psychosocial factors associated with substance abuse, multiple concerns exist in the newborn period, including:

- Alterations in infant–parent attachment
- Newborn safety issues

- Exposure to secondhand smoke
- Infant mental health issues
- Exposure to domestic violence

Treatment Measures for Infants With NAS

Tests that may be done to diagnose withdrawal in a newborn include:

- Recommended treatment is based on the type of drug used, infant's overall health and transition, and gestational age at the time of birth
- NAS scoring assessment should be performed, which assigns points based on each symptom and its severity and helps determine treatment course
- Toxicology screen of first bowel movements (meconium)
- Drug screening via urinalysis
- Some infants may require medication for withdrawal
- High-calorie formula may be needed

INFANTS BORN ON THE THRESHOLD OF VIABILITY

The threshold of viability takes into account gestational age at the time of birth and birth weight. The combination of these factors can drastically affect morbidity and mortality (Tables 8.1 and 8.2). Although these infants may survive, they are at risk for long-term disabilities, including:

- Psychomotor disabilities
- Neuromuscular disabilities
- Mental disabilities
- Sensory disabilities
- Communication-related disabilities
- Cerebral palsy

TABLE 8.1 Survival Rates Associated With Completed Gestational Weeks

Completed Gestational Weeks	Survival Rate (%)
21	0
22	21
23	30
24	50
25	75
26	80
27	90
> 28	> 90

Data obtained from Lemons et al. (2001).

TABLE 8.2 Infant Survival by Birth Weight

Birth Weight (g)	Survival Rate (%)
400–500	11
501–600	31
601–700	62
701–800	75
801–900	88
901–1,000	90
> 1,000	> 92

Data obtained from Lemons et al. (2001).

Outcomes Associated With Aggressive Neonatal Intensive Care Unit Care

Newborns weighing between 500 and 750 g are at risk for the following adverse outcomes:

- Growth failure
- Intraventricular hemorrhage

- Respiratory distress syndrome
- Chronic lung disease
- Severe brain injury (intraventricular hemorrhage and periventricular leukomalacia)
- Necrotizing enterocolitis
- Nosocomial infections
- Retinopathy of prematurity
- Cerebral palsy
- Vision impairment
- Hearing loss

Evaluating Infant Status at Birth

Newborns born on the threshold of viability should be assessed and care decisions should be made based on the following:

- Gestational age
- Birth weight
- Condition at time of birth
- Morbidity and mortality data and statistics
- Newborn's response to resuscitative and stabilizing measures
- Parental preferences
- Knowledge that care plan may change based on newborn's condition
- Withdrawal of life support may be warranted if deterioration of condition occurs

Ethical Implications

Occasionally there are ethical and legal implications that may impact the care of an infant born on the threshold of viability. These issues should be addressed using a systematic approach:

- Parents should be counseled on probable outcomes and options and be involved in decision making.

- Family-centered collaborative decision making takes into account the interests of all family members.
- Physicians/care providers must respond to an infant's life-threatening conditions by providing treatment (including appropriate nutrition, hydration, and medication), which in the treating physician's reasonable medical judgment will be most likely to be effective in ameliorating or correcting all such conditions.
- Care can be withheld if the newborn is:
  - Irreversibly comatose
  - Treatment is only prolonging death
  - Treatment is futile for survival
- When disagreements in appropriate care measures exist, each state's child protection agency provides jurisdiction for decision making.
- Infant Care Review Committees (Infant Bioethics Committees) should be formed and used to guide complex decisions.

FAST FACTS in a NUTSHELL

In 1995, neonatal care guidelines became law under the Federal Child Abuse Law.

NEONATAL ANESTHESIA AND SURGERY

Surgery in the neonatal period is only performed when absolutely necessary. Anesthesia use carries some risks and requires careful monitoring by an experienced clinician. Commonly used anesthetic agents include inhaled anesthesia and regional anesthesia. The conditions that most commonly require surgical procedures during the neonatal period include:

- Tracheoesophageal fistula
- Gastroschisis

- Omphalocele
- Encephalocoele
- Pyloric stenosis
- Congenital diaphragmatic hernia
- Imperforate anus
- Ventriculoperitoneal shunt
- Cardiac cauterization
- Posterior urethral valve excision

Consideration for Neonates Receiving Anesthesia and Undergoing Surgery

- Intraoperative fluid management
- Management of apnea
- Transitional circulation can reoccur
- Adequate ventilation during surgery
- Management of blood loss
- Maintaining glucose levels
- Temperature maintenance
- Existence of coagulopathies
- Risk of infection
- Pain management in the postoperative period
- Risk for anesthesia toxicity

NEONATAL TRANSPORT

Neonatal transport is sometimes warranted if an infant requires care or surgical intervention that is not available at the delivering facility. U.S. hospitals have three levels of nursery units, although some regions will designate hospitals based on a four-tier division:

- Well baby (Level I neonatal intensive care unit [NICU])
  - Newborns born after 35 weeks
  - Newborns in stable condition

- Special Care Nursery (Level II NICU)
  - Newborns born beyond 32 weeks
  - Provides monitoring after birth
  - Intravenous fluids and medications
  - Temperature stability
  - Premature infants
  - Jaundice
- Level III NICU
  - Care for any gestational age
  - Provides respiratory support
  - Intravenous fluids and medications
  - Tube feedings
- Level IV NICU
  - Care of threshold-of-viability newborns
  - Intensive respiratory support
  - Neonatal surgery

Perinatal Regionalization System

Perinatal regionalization is a system designating where infants are born or are transferred after birth based on the amount of care that they need. In regionalized systems, very ill or very small infants are placed in facilities that provide the highest level of care with high-level technology and specialized health providers on site. Whenever possible, mothers are sent to the most appropriate medical facility to care for the needs of the newborn prior to delivery; however, not all pregnant women can be safely transferred prior to birth and neonatal transfer may be needed.

Essential Skills of the Neonatal Transport Team

Neonates may need immediate transfer upon delivery to obtain the most appropriate care. Transport can include ground, helicopter, or airplane transport options. During transport, stabilization, therapeutic hypothermia, ventilation, continuous monitoring, and drug administration may be needed. Nurses on neonatal transport teams need to provide precise critical thinking skills and possess extensive clinical expertise.

9

Families Facing Life-Altering Situations

In the United States, there are almost 4 million births each year. Of these, 2.7% (15,000/yr) will have birth defects incompatible with life (Centers for Disease Control and Prevention, 2013b). Many, but not all, of these defects are known prior to birth. Families faced with giving birth to a newborn with a birth defect that is incompatible with life experience intense emotional responses and need extensive support and education to deal with their loss.

Other families may experience horrific birth trauma that leaves a newborn with lifelong adverse health consequences. These families need support, education, and comprehensive resources to provide the best possible care to their newborn.

Nurses dealing with the complex ethical, emotional, and legal issues related to the unique needs of this population need to possess a thorough understanding of these challenging situations and the issues that will likely impact the care they provide to the newborn and family.

During this part of the orientation, the nurse will be able to:

1. Identify lethal anomalies that are considered incompatible with life
2. Describe the phases of grief and how they impact grieving parents

3. Analyze the needs of families following a neonatal death
4. List the most frequent ethical issues encountered when caring for newborns
5. Summarize care needs for newborns who have experienced a birth injury

NEWBORNS WITH LETHAL ANOMALIES

Anomalies that are not compatible with life will result in newborn death. Of infants born with lethal anomalies, 75% will die within 10 days of life, with 90% dying within 4 months of birth. Diagnosis of lethal anomalies typically occurs during the prenatal period, although the possibility of a missed diagnosis or lack of prenatal care may lead to undetected anomalies that are not identified until birth. Routine prenatal tools that typically identify these anomalies include:

- First trimester screening (ultrasound examination for nuchal translucency testing with maternal blood screening)
- Ultrasound
- Chronic villus sampling
- Amniocentesis
- Fetal echocardiography
- Quadruple screen

Types of Birth Defects Considered Lethal Anomalies

Lethal anomalies are those that are considered incompatible with life. The most common defects include:

- Anencephaly
- Trisomy 13
- Trisomy 18
- Renal agenesis
- Thanatophoric dysplasia
- Alobar holoprosencephaly
- Certain types of hydrocephalic cases
- Certain hypoplastic cardiac conditions (when heart transplant is not a treatment option)

Pregnancy Options for Birth Defects Incompatible With Life

When a lethal birth defect is identified, extensive counseling is warranted. Families are generally given the following pregnancy options:

- Continuation of pregnancy in a supportive manner with no planned life-saving interventions at birth
- Continuation of pregnancy with life-saving measures provided at birth
- Elective termination of pregnancy

The following care measures are imperative:

- Complete explanation of diagnosis, prognosis, and anticipated outcomes
- Referral to genetic specialist/perinatologist
- Discussion of each pregnancy option
- Information that infants with the identified diagnosis have rarely survived
- Provide life expectancy averages
- Honest prognosis of surviving infants with vast medical complications
- Assist with second opinion per parent request
- Risk of reoccurrence with future pregnancies
- Referral to child life specialist to help with sibling preparation
- Bereavement support and planning should begin at time of diagnosis.

FAST FACTS in a NUTSHELL

Although Internet-based resources can provide support and valuable information, be aware that anecdotes about "miracles" posted on blogs and other Internet sites can sometimes lead to unreasonable expectations and further pain.

Nursing Care to Families Facing a Birth Defect Incompatible With Life

Care measures include holistic care based on the selected pregnancy option. Each family needs specific, individualized, holistic nursing care regardless of the pregnancy option they choose.

Continuation of Pregnancy

Continuation of a pregnancy following prenatal diagnosis of a lethal anomaly occurs in 18% of women (Courtwright, Laughon, & Doron, 2011). Appropriate care measures are needed to ensure supportive, family-centered care, including:

- Ongoing prenatal care with a perinatologist
- Frequent ultrasound monitoring
- Monitoring for maternal complications
- Referral for counseling and psychological support
- Family support, including support groups and peer support
- Preparation on expectations of infant appearance, birth process, and anticipated outcomes at time of birth
- Assistance with sibling education and support
- Assistance with detailed birth plan based on family's preferences
  - Desired interventions/lack of interventions at time of birth
  - Identification of support persons to be present during labor and birth
  - Postbirth family/sibling visitation
  - Planned newborn interactions following live birth (holding infant, breastfeeding infant, dressing newborn, sibling/extended family member visit, spending time with infant alone, pain control for newborn)
  - Desired interaction with newborn following death (holding infant, keeping infant at bedside for certain period of time, visit from extended family/siblings, religious ceremonies)

  - Predetermined plan on notifying friends/family of birth outcomes after delivery
  - Postdelivery support plan (clergy, support groups, funeral home arrangements)
- Memory box
- Consultation with grief counselor
- Contingency plan of care for newborns who exceed expected life expectancy period
- Plan of care with life expectancies more than several days
  - Discharge home
  - Palliative care
  - Perinatal hospice referral
- Autopsy
- Assist with identifying resources for final arrangements

FAST FACTS in a NUTSHELL

Families that make comprehensive plans for the newborn's birth and death feel a sense of control during the labor, birth, and postpartum periods. Creating a detailed birth, life, and death plan can empower parents during this time of intense grief.

Termination of Pregnancy

- Method of termination is dependent on gestational age at time of termination
- Education on procedure, expectations, and appearance of infant following delivery
- Psychological support
- Birth plan
  - Presence of support persons
  - Postbirth interaction with infant (holding infant; dressing infant; photos; visitation of extended family members; support persons, including clergy, grief counselor)
  - Autopsy and final arrangements
- Assist with identifying resources for final arrangements

> Parents should be counseled to use caution with how much information is shared with others and limit specific information sharing to friends and family who will offer support and acceptance. Discordant opinions can cause pain, guilt, and additional stress.

NEWBORN DEATH AND DYING

Each year, 19,000 newborns die in the neonatal period. The leading causes of neonatal death include:

- Premature birth
- Congenital heart defects
- Lung defects
- Chromosomal/genetic defects
- Brain and central nervous system defects

Phases of Grief

Psychologically, maternal–infant (parent–infant) attachment begins during pregnancy, as parents have dreams of what their baby will be like. Intrauterine loss or newborn loss is a loss of personhood for that child, no matter how long the life lasted. When parents are informed that their newborn will likely die in utero or shortly after birth, multiple intense psychological reactions occur, including disbelief, profound grief, guilt regarding diagnosis (self-blame), guilt regarding termination of pregnancy, fear of not being able to have a healthy child, and fear that their other children could have a child with the same diagnosis. Families experience the following stages of grief:

- Denial (shock, disbelief)
- Anger (self-directed, spouse, God, health care providers)

- Bargaining (wanting more time, prolonging the inevitable loss)
- Depression (crying, withdrawal, increased risk of postpartum mood and anxiety disorders)
- Acceptance (coming to terms with the diagnosis/loss can take months or years)

Nursing Care of the Family Experiencing a Neonatal Death

- Assist with tasks of grieving
- Provide privacy
- Provide explanation of etiology
- Provide time with newborn and allow personalized interactions based on parental requests/wishes
- Provide appropriate referrals
  - Clergy, religious support per family request
  - Grief counselor or social worker
  - Support groups, peer support
  - Genetic counselor for future pregnancy planning
- Memory box
- Autopsy and consent forms
- Follow up with cards, phone calls, and other supportive care measures after discharge
- Screen for postpartum mood and anxiety disorders

═══════════════════════ *FAST FACTS in a NUTSHELL*

Nurses Should Provide the 3 H's Following Any Neonatal Death: Hug, Hush, and Hang Around
Now I Lay Me Down to Sleep (NILMDTS) is an invaluable gift of remembrance photography for parents suffering the loss of a newborn/stillborn. Comprised of volunteer photographers, NILMDTS will come to the hospital at any time, day or night, to capture the fleeting moments of a preterm/critically ill newborn's life on film. The service is provided free of charge to the parents.

COMPLEX ETHICAL AND LEGAL DECISION MAKING

Parents and health care providers face a number of complex ethical issues regarding decision making for infants with conditions incompatible with life and those with life-threatening or lethal anomalies. Common ethical issues and decisions include:

- Withholding or withdrawing life support
- Do not resuscitate (DNR) orders
- DNR before cardiopulmonary resuscitation (CPR)
- CPR withheld
- No delivery room resuscitation
- Mechanical ventilation withheld
- Mechanical ventilation withdrawn

Nurse's Role When Facing Complex Ethical Issues

- Examine one's own beliefs about complex ethical issues.
- Never place one's own beliefs above the patient.
- Accept one's own personal grief regarding the care of the family.
- Do not voice personal beliefs or provide judgments about parental decision making.
- Provide supportive, compassionate care to all families regardless of your own beliefs.
- Decision making and clinical care plans should be made based on the basis of fact, current research, and evidenced-based practice.
- Provide parents with complete disclosure of information.
- Encourage the hospital to develop a Futility Policy for Newborn Care.
- Consult an ethicist or ethics committee for guidance in complex ethical situations.

- Provide ongoing support and education for the family, regardless of the family's socioeconomic status, personal character, or source of illness.
- Respect cultural, family, and religious beliefs.

CARING FOR FAMILIES WITH NEONATAL BIRTH INJURIES

Although the majority of births are uneventful, 0.1% of births result in adverse outcomes that are related to delivery, which then result in a birth injury. Birth injuries can occur as a result of:

- Hypoxia
- Asphyxia
- Birth trauma
- Prolapsed cord
- Delayed cesarean section
- Maternal complications
- Nonreassuring fetal status
- Physician/provider malpractice or negligence
- Complications during cesarean birth
- Errors or complications from instrument deliveries

Clinical complications related to birth injuries may include:

- Cerebral palsy
- Dislocations
- Erb's palsy
- Spinal cord injuries
- Nasal septal dislocation
- Ocular injuries
- Intracranial hemorrhage
- Neurological injuries
- Abdominal injuries
- Instrument-related injuries (lacerations, fractures, nerve damage)

Nursing Considerations for Newborns With Birth Injuries

- Identify maternal risk factors
  - Maternal obesity
  - Macrosomia
  - Cesarean birth
  - Maternal pelvic abnormalities
  - Abnormal fetal presentation
  - Instrument-assisted birth
- Provide physical examination to assess for injuries
- Obtain appropriate diagnostic testing
- Referral to specialist related to specific injury (orthopedic surgeon, neurologist, etc.)
- Acknowledge parents' emotional reactions
  - Disbelief
  - Denial
  - Anger
  - Guilt
  - Sadness
- Provide referrals to support groups, peer support programs, or to a parent with similar experiences
- Offer pastoral/clergy support
- Obtain social work consult
- Provide honest, straightforward information

FAST FACTS in a NUTSHELL

Nurses should never provide inaccurate information or attempt to cover up a situation when malpractice or negligence exists following a birth injury. Ethical principles that guide nursing practice should never be compromised.

10

Discharge and Health-Promotion Teaching for Parents

For new parents, leaving the health care setting can create mixed feelings. Parents need extensive teaching prior to discharge in order to learn how to adequately and safely provide for their newborn. Ongoing well-baby visits and immunizations are imperative for the newborn to ensure proper growth, development, and optimal health. Newborn and infant health-promotion counseling is an important part of discharge education and is almost exclusively performed by nursing staff. The nurse needs to provide information in a variety of ways to meet the specific learning needs of different parents. By assessing different learning styles and needs, education levels, reading abilities, language barriers, and the presence of disabilities that could impact comprehension, the nurse can provide essential teaching using a variety of teaching strategies.

During this part of the orientation, the nurse will be able to:

1. List the appropriate intervals for routine well-baby visits during the first month of life
2. Discuss strategies to reduce parental refusal of immunizations
3. Describe the components of safety that are necessary to perform newborn bathing and nail care
4. Identify symptoms of umbilical cord infection

5. Discuss normal newborn temperature assessment and how to properly maintain the thermal environment for newborns
6. List normal newborn voiding and stool patterns
7. Delineate normal sleep patterns for newborns
8. Describe normal crying patterns and interventions to reduce crying

EQUIPMENT

Measuring tape, scale, growth charts.

WELL-BABY VISITS

Components of well-baby visits include examination and evaluation of the following:

- Weight
- Length
- Abdominal circumference
- Head circumference
- Evaluation of appropriate growth and development
- Physical examination
- Parental education
  - Safety
  - Ongoing identification of risk factors
  - Risk-reduction strategies
  - Health-promotion strategies

FAST FACTS in a NUTSHELL

Although the outpatient newborn exam typically occurs within 2 to 5 days after birth, parents should be taught to seek medical attention earlier if a complication or unexpected event occurs.

Newborn Examinations

The newborn should be seen within 2 to 5 days of birth (Table 10.1) and again between 1 and 4 weeks. Essential

TABLE 10.1 Assessment Data and Parent Teaching for Newborn Well Visits

Age	Age-Specific Assessment Data	Parent Teaching
2–5 days	• Weight loss/gain/presence of abnormal vomiting or other gastrointestinal issues • Infant feeding method • Frequency of voiding and stooling • Safety measures being used (not leaving infant unattended where falls could occur, leaving infant with appropriate caretakers, providing infant with appropriate nutrition, ensuring safe environment free from environmental hazards). • Volume of milk consumption to determine whether vitamin D supplementation is needed • Use of infant care seat and current position • Sleep positions • Smoke/carbon monoxide detectors in home • Hepatitis B vaccination status	• Normal newborn growth and development • Breastfeeding frequency/duration • Problems/concerns related to breastfeeding • Pumping and breast-milk storage • Safety issues related to formula preparation • Safe sleeping positions (Back to Sleep positioning) • Normal infant sleep patterns • Crying patterns • Safety issues (fall prevention, possible choking risks, suffocation hazards, car seat use, safe water temperature) • Participation in an infant cardiopulmonary resuscitation course • Assess for maternal postpartum depression and mood disorders • Abusive head trauma (AHT) • Illness prevention/handwashing • Prevention of AHT • Importance of immunizations • Sunburn prevention
1–4 weeks	• Feeding difficulties • Inadequate weight gain • Cord condition/cord site	• Crying/colic • Bathing • Illness prevention/handwashing • Car safety • Ways to soothe baby • Prevention of AHT • Future immunizations • Sunburn prevention

components of those visits should include evaluation of the following:

- Evaluation of feeding
- Weight gain/loss
- Adjustment to parenthood
- Identification of specific parental concerns
- Safety

The hepatitis B immunization is generally given prior to discharge from the medical facility. Infant immunizations typically begin at 2 months; however, education on the importance of immunizations should begin at the initial newborn visits. For families traveling out of the country, the Centers for Disease Control and Prevention (CDC) recommends certain immunizations.

Family and Environmental Risk Factors

Certain risk factors are also important to assess because they can put the infant at risk for adverse health outcomes:

- Family risk factors
  - History of intimate partner violence or domestic violence
  - History of past child abuse or child neglect
  - Low level of parental education achievement
  - Low socioeconomic status/poverty
  - Adolescent parents
  - Severe parental mental illness
  - Parental substance abuse
  - Parents who oppose/decline immunizations
  - Presence of stressful life events within the family
  - Low parental IQ
  - Lack of maternal–infant attachment
- Environmental risk factors
  - Lack of family/community support
  - Lack of access to health care
  - Rural geographic location
  - Crowded living conditions

- Exposure to secondhand smoke
- Enrollment in low-quality child care

========================== *FAST FACTS in a NUTSHELL*

Infants exposed to secondhand smoke are more likely to experience allergies, asthma, and hospitalizations during the first year of life.

Well visits should be scheduled at regular intervals:

- 2 to 5 days after birth
- 1 to 4 weeks
- 2 months
- 4 months
- 6 months
- 9 months
- 12 months

Immunization Schedule

Immunizations are an important measure that can dramatically reduce childhood and community illness. Immunizations begin at birth (hepatitis B) and continue throughout childhood. Appendix A includes the CDC vaccination guidelines.

Recommended Immunizations for Overseas Travel

Infants traveling outside of the United States are particularly vulnerable for infectious disease because of their immature immune systems and lack of adequate vaccinations due to their young age. Overseas travel requires preplanning and specific interventions to ensure infant safety. Parents should be advised to:

- Consult a travel immunization specialist to determine which specific vaccines are needed for the country of travel.
- Consult the pediatrician 3 to 4 months ahead of travel to initiate an accelerated vaccine schedule.

- If possible, travel should be delayed until infant is 9 months of age, when yellow fever vaccine can be given.
- All infants should receive meningococcal meningitis vaccine prior to any overseas travel.
- Counsel parents that some vaccines cannot be given early.
- Breastfeeding is the safest feeding choice.
- If formula is used, parents should bring formula with them and only use purified water to mix the formula.

Parental Refusal of Immunizations

Approximately 6% of parents refuse vaccinations, whereas another 13% delay vaccinations (Harrington, 2011). Parents refuse or delay immunizations for a number of reasons (Figure 10.1):

- Belief that diseases vaccine guards against have been eradicated
- Concerns over vaccine safety
- Belief that multiple vaccines overload the immune system
- Belief that vaccines are associated with autism
- Belief that ingredients found in vaccines (thimerosal and aluminum salts) are dangerous
- Believe their child has a medical condition that makes vaccinations dangerous
- Personal, philosophical, or religious beliefs

Counseling for Parents Refusing Immunizations (Harrington, 2011)

- Begin discussing vaccination information at initial visit
- Provide factual information in a respectful, nonpatronizing, and nonconfrontational manner
- Provide vaccination information sheets at least 1 month prior to the scheduled immunization
- Discuss need to prevent community outbreaks
- Direct parents to credible websites
- Be respectful of parents' authority

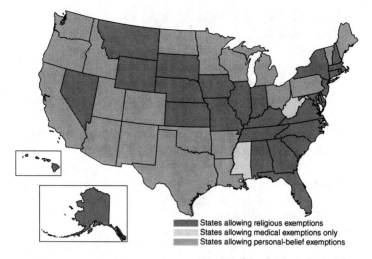

FIGURE 10.1 State exemption status for immunizations.
Source: Centers for Disease Control and Prevention (2013d).

- Provide sucrose administration and swaddling as pain reduction mechanisms during injections
- Ongoing refusal warrants appropriate interactions
  - Completion of the American Academy of Pediatrics Refusal-to-Vaccinate form
  - Notification of office/clinic policies if refusal warrants patient dismissal from practice

Bathing

Bathing in the newborn period should begin with sponge bathing until the umbilical cord falls off completely. Sponge bathing can be performed every 2 to 3 days, or more frequently in summer months as needed. Parents should be taught the following for sponge bathing:

- Obtain all supplies prior to starting the bath (washcloth, towels, soap).
- Place infant on a surface that can support the infant and hold supplies.
- Never leave infant unattended during bath.
- Obtain a bowl of water.

- Undress infant and keep covered with a towel to prevent heat loss.
- Use a small amount of mild cleanser that is free of fragrance and dye, tearless, and pH neutral.
- Dry each body area to prevent heat loss.
- Never hold infant under running water, as temperature changes can occur.
- Review a systematic method for bathing, starting with the eyes, face, and progressing downward.
- The genitals should be cleaned last, prior to washing the hair.
- Once the body has been bathed, infants can be swaddled so hair can be washed.

Tub Baths and Showering

- Tub baths should not be started until the umbilical cord has completely fallen off.
- Obtain all needed equipment.
- Test water to ensure proper temperature prior to placing infant in tub.
- Support of the head and body are needed.
- Never leave child unattended to answer the phone, door, check on other children, etc.
- Parents wishing to shower infants during their own shower should be counseled on safety issues.
- Newborns should never be taken into hot tubs or saunas due to extreme temperatures.

Skin and Nail Care

- Never cut nails in the hospital setting prior to discharge due to risk of nosocomial infection.
- Parents may file or cut nails with infant-size nail clippers.
- Cutting nails after a bath can soften nails.
- If skin is nicked or cut during trimming, keep area clean and watch for signs of infection (uncommon).
- Baby powder should never be used because the particles can cause respiratory issues

- Lotion and creams are generally not needed; if used, one designed for infants should be used sparingly.
- Avoid direct sunlight and damaging rays; keep baby in shaded area or in stroller.
- If absolutely necessary, apply a small amount of SPF 30 sunscreen after testing on the wrist prior to application.

Cord Care and Assessment

- Cords typically continue to dry for 7 to 21 days before falling off.
- A small wound may be present at the site and will heal within a few days.
- Cord should be kept clean and dry.
- Diapers should be folded underneath the cord.
- One-piece outfits should be avoided until the cord falls off.
- Signs of infection warrant immediate evaluation: fever; cord or surrounding area becomes red, warm, or edematous; foul-smelling odor from cord; pus; active bleeding.
- Umbilical granulomas (areas that do not heal) should be reported to the pediatrician.

Maintaining an Appropriate Thermal Environment at Home

- Temperature setting between 68° F to 72° F for winter and 75° F to 78° F for summer
- Avoid fans, drafty areas, open windows, and direct access to heat/air conditioning sources
- Do not overbundle/overdress newborn, as this increases risk of sudden infant death syndrome.
- Sleep in light-weight, single-layer item that would be comfortable for adult in same room
- Infant should not feel hot to touch or be perspiring profusely.
- In higher temperatures, baby requires increased fluid consumption to prevent dehydration.
- In colder temperatures, extra layers may be needed to prevent chilling.

Temperature Variations and Symptoms Related to Illness

- Normal temperature is 97°F to 100.3°F (rectal)
- Presence of fever or low temperature can indicate infection
- Fevers in newborns and infants less than 3 months are cause for concern
- Lethargy is an important sign of illness

Reasons to Seek Medical Attention

- Fever exceeds 100.4°F in newborn/infant less than 3 months
- Lethargy
- Refusal to feed
- Cough
- Signs of an earache (pulling on ear)
- Unusual fussiness or sleepiness
- Vomiting
- Diarrhea (more than 1 occurrence per hour, blood in the stool)
- Hard stools with straining and no bowel movement for 3 days
- Seizures
- Less than four wet diapers per day
- Dehydration (dry mouth, less than four wet diapers/day, sunken soft spot, lack of tears, irritability)
- More than two green watery stools in a 24-hour period

════════════════════════════*FAST FACTS in a NUTSHELL*

Parents should be encouraged to call their health care provider immediately when in doubt regarding an illness in their newborn. Stress to parents that it is better to call and receive reassurance than not call and have a critical emergency occur.

Normal Urinary and Stooling Patterns

- Infants should void within 24 hours of birth.
- After 10 days, colorless, odorless urine is excreted up to 15 times per day.
- Initially, multiple stools are excreted each day.
- After 2 weeks of age, stooling may become less frequent.
- Breastfed infants tend to have multiple loose, mustard-colored stools with sour-milk smell several times each day.
- Formula-fed infants tend to have brown, semi-formed stools that are firm and pasty with a foul odor, which can occur every day to every other day.
- Grunting or turning red during stooling is normal and not a sign of constipation.
- Constipation is marked by hard stools and straining.
- Diarrhea stools are frequent, loose, and watery and may result in a foul-smelling odor.

Normal Newborn Sleep Habits

- Total sleep 16 to 17 hours per day
- Sleeps for periods of 2 to 4 hours at a time
- Increased time spent in rapid-eye-movement sleep, which is lighter and more easily disturbed
- At 2 weeks of age, begin distinguishing night and day and encouraging nighttime sleeping.
  - Active when awake during the day
  - Keep rooms brightly lit
  - Wake for all feedings
  - Do not attempt to reduce normal household noise
  - At night, do not wake for feedings
  - Do not engage in play or talk excessively with newborn at night
  - Keep lights dim and room quiet
  - Put back to sleep after each feeding
  - Establish bedtime rituals (changing into night clothes, singing, kissing goodnight)
- Never administer over-the-counter or home remedies for sleeping.

Crying Behaviors

- Vary from infant to infant, from virtually none to frequent crying episodes
- Increase at about 2 weeks after birth
- Peak at 6 weeks
- Decrease gradually until stable at 3 to 4 months of age
- One fussy period per day is common

Common Causes for Crying

- Hunger
- Gastrointestinal reflux disease
- Flatus
- Food intolerances in maternal diet associated with breastfeeding
- Colic
- Illness

Interventions for Parents of Crying Newborns

- Respond quickly to crying.
- Look for hunger cues (awake state, lip smacking, rooting, putting hands in the mouth).
- Breastfeed baby on demand.
- Burp newborn after feeding.
- Place over your lap on abdomen and gently rub back.
- Check environmental factors to rule out whether newborn is too hot or too cold.
- Assess for fever, lethargy, and signs of illness.
- Change diaper.
- Encourage sleep.
- Avoid letting infant become overtired.
- Carrying and holding newborns reduces crying.

II

Promoting Healthy Families in the Community

Promotion of health and wellness for the newborn and infant begins immediately following birth and continues into the first year of life. Nurses play a crucial role in providing parental education for injury and illness prevention by providing education about infant injuries. By identifying parents at risk, additional support and interventions can be implemented to support families with limited resources.

Community-based postpartum services provide families with invaluable resources to promote health and family wellness. The nurse provides these resources during the postpartum period and at well visits during the first year of life. The health and well-being of infants and children are closely associated with maternal mental health and well-being. Postpartum depression and mood disorder screening are imperative, as 15% to 20% of women develop postpartum depression after the birth of an infant (Davidson, 2012).

Some women will leave the hospital facility without their infants due to prematurity and newborn illness or congenital birth defects. Others will relinquish their infants or leave without a live baby as a result of fetal demise. These women have unique care needs that warrant specialized nursing care and support.

During this part of the orientation, the nurse will be able to:

1. Define sudden unexpected infant death (SUID)
2. List the most common causes of infant injuries in the first year of life
3. Describe interventions to reduce the risk of sudden infant death syndrome (SIDS)
4. Identify the symptoms associated with postpartum depression
5. Delineate supportive care measures that can be used for the woman who leaves the hospital without her infant
6. Describe types of community-based support systems for new families

SUDDEN UNEXPECTED INFANT DEATH

SUID is the death of an infant less than 1 year of age that occurs suddenly and unexpectedly. After investigation, these deaths may be diagnosed as suffocation, asphyxia, entrapment, infection, ingestions, metabolic diseases, cardiac arrhythmias, trauma (accidental or nonaccidental), or SIDS.

UNINTENTIONAL INJURIES LEADING TO INFANT DEATH

Unintentional injuries are the fifth-leading cause of death in infants less than 1 year of age. The most common causes of unintentional infant deaths include the following:

- Infant suffocation
- Motor vehicle-, traffic-related
- Drowning
- Fire/burns
- Poisoning
- Falls
- Other transportation-related sources

- Avoid having infant sleep in bed with others.
- Remove extra blankets, pillows, heavy comforters, or toys in crib.
- Always secure infant in rear-facing car seat.
- Ensure home has functioning smoke detectors.
- Test smoke detectors each month.
- Never hold infant while cooking.
- Never leave child unattended in a pool or area containing standing water.
- Never leave an infant on a bed or other elevated surface unattended.
- Use infant gates, window guards, and stair gates to prevent falls.
- Never leave medications in reach of children.
- Dispose of all old medications that are no longer in use.
- Keep all medication in containers with safety tops.
- Make sure food items are properly cut to correct size to prevent choking.

ABUSIVE HEAD TRAUMA

Abusive head trauma (AHT), also known as *shaken baby syndrome*, occurs as a result of direct blows to the head, dropping or throwing a child, or shaking a child. Head trauma is the leading cause of death in child-abuse cases in the United States. Although any infant can sustain AHT, it occurs more frequently in low-socioeconomic-status families with male infants. Perpetrators are often male caregivers who react as a result of the infant crying.

Symptoms of AHT may include:

- Lethargy
- Irritability
- Vomiting
- Poor sucking or swallowing
- Decreased appetite
- Lack of smiling or vocalizing

- Rigidity
- Seizures
- Difficulty breathing
- Altered consciousness
- Unequal pupil size
- Hemorrhages in the retinas of the eyes
- Skull fractures
- Swelling of the brain
- Subdural hematomas
- Rib and long-bone fractures
- Bruises around the head, neck, or chest
- Inability to lift the head
- Inability to focus the eyes or track movement

Adverse Outcomes Related to AHT

AHT can result in immediate death for the infant. Adverse outcomes related to AHT in infants who survive include:

- Partial or total blindness
- Hearing loss
- Seizures
- Developmental delays
- Intellectual disability
- Speech and learning difficulties
- Problems with memory and attention
- Severe intellectual impairment
- Cerebral palsy

FAST FACTS in a NUTSHELL

If an infant is ever experiencing any symptoms of AHT, immediate medical attention is imperative.

Certain parents are at risk for committing child abuse and warrant ongoing assessment after birth. Resources for these parents can reduce the risk of AHT and other forms of child abuse. At-risk parents include:

- Teen parents
- Parents who were abused as children
- Parents with other children in state custody or living with relatives
- Intimate partner violence in the home
- Drug or alcohol abuse
- Mental health and pre-existing medical issues
- History of neglect
- Lack of knowledge of infant behavior and child development
- Single parenthood
- Low education levels
- Low socioeconomic status
- Large number of young children in family
- Nonbiological transient caregivers

Strategies to Reduce Child Abuse

- Home visits for at-risk families
- Public awareness
- Parenting classes
- Support groups for new parents
- Peer mentoring programs
- Substance-abuse programs for parents
- Respite care for parents of disabled infants
- Family resource centers in low-income areas

11. PROMOTING HEALTHY FAMILIES IN THE COMMUNITY

If child abuse is ever suspected, it should be immediately reported to the county social services agency. Nurses and other health care professionals are considered mandatory reporters and must by law report suspected abuse.

SUDDEN INFANT DEATH SYNDROME

SIDS is the sudden death of an infant less than 1 year of age that cannot be explained after a thorough investigation, autopsy, death-scene investigation, and a review of the clinical history has been performed. It is estimated that there are 2,100 SIDS deaths annually in the United States (Centers for Disease Control and Prevention [CDC], 2013e). Blacks and American Indian/Alaskan Natives have double the risk of SIDS (CDC, 2013e).

Prevention Strategies for SIDS

- Place baby on his or her back to sleep.
- Use a firm sleep surface covered by a fitted sheet.
- Baby should sleep in a crib.
- Cosleeping should be discouraged.
- Soft objects, toys, and loose bedding should not be placed in crib.
- Secondhand smoke should be avoided completely.
- Breastfeeding during the first year reduces SIDS risk.
- Provide a pacifier that is not attached to a string.
- Avoid overheating the room temperature and overheating the infant by overdressing.

SCREENING AND PREVENTION OF POSTPARTUM DEPRESSION

Postpartum depression affects 15% to 20% of new mothers. Other postpartum mood and anxiety disorders include postpartum anxiety, postpartum obsessive-compulsive disorder, and postpartum psychosis. Symptoms of postpartum depression vary, but diagnosis is based on the presence of five or more of the following symptoms:

- Depressed mood
- Loss of interest in previously enjoyed activities
- Significant weight loss or appetite change
- Insomnia or hypersomnia
- Loss of energy or fatigue
- Feelings of worthlessness or excessive guilt
- Diminished ability to concentrate
- Suicidal thoughts

Risk Factors for Postpartum Mood Disorders

There are multiple risk factors for postpartum mood disorders; therefore, it is important to identify women at risk so proper screening can be performed. Women with bipolar disorder are at greatest risk of developing postpartum psychosis and need additional support and assessment during the postpartum period. Risk factors for postpartum mood disorders include:

- Past history of mental health disorder (especially depression)
- Past history of postpartum depression
- Isolation
- Poor social support
- Other stressors (moving, job loss, pregnancy complications, etc.)
- Financial problems
- Marital/relationship issues

Nursing Interventions for Postpartum Mood Disorders

- Postpartum depression screening should be performed on all women at the postpartum visit.

- Pediatric care providers can also screen women for postpartum mood disorders, because they often have prolonged contact with women after the birth.
- Facilities should select a screening tool/instrument for routine use, such as:
  - Edinburgh Postpartum Depression Scale (EPDS)
  - Postpartum Depression Screening Scale (PDSS)
  - Patient Health Questionnaire (PHQ-9)
  - Center for Epidemiologic Studies Depression Scale (CES-D)
- Encourage participation in postpartum and new-mother support groups.
- Refer to postpartum depression support groups.
- Refer to Postpartum Support International.
- Interdisciplinary care management
  - Psychological counseling
  - Medication evaluation
  - Support groups
  - Peer support

POSTPARTUM SUPPORT SERVICES

The postpartum period represents a time of tremendous change for the new family. Adequate postpartum services are needed to ensure optimal newborn and family well-being. Families that receive postpartum support services have better outcomes, reduce the risk of maternal postpartum mood disorders, and are more likely to act appropriately if newborn complications occur. Suggested community-based services should include:

- Social support in the postpartum period
- New mother/infant support classes in the community
- Postpartum depression groups
- Breastfeeding consultation services

- Breastfeeding support services (La Leche League)
- Support services for new fathers
- Telephone follow-up from care providers
- More frequent visits for at-risk mothers
- Availability of use of online support and services
- Interdisciplinary care services
- Social services support
- Low-income clinics

DISCHARGE OF THE MOTHER WITHOUT HER INFANT

The majority of infants are discharged with their parents; however, a small number of women will be discharged without their infants. In most cases, the infant remains hospitalized due to illness or prematurity. A small number of women place their infants for adoption, whereas others have had social services intervention that has prohibited the release of the newborn with the mother. Other women may have suffered a fetal demise or neonatal loss, which is discussed in detail in Chapter 9.

Considerations for Women Discharged Without Their Infants

- Psychological implications (sadness, guilt, fear, depression)
- Physical demands for the mother (traveling back and forth to the hospital, pumping breast milk around the clock)
- Supporting the mother with a hospitalized infant
  - Encourage frequent visits.
  - Encourage phone calls to check on infant's status.
  - Support breastfeeding efforts.

- Facilitate sibling interactions and visitation.
- Provide an area for parents to rest and sleep.
- Supporting the mother who relinquishes her infant
  - Provide mementos, including a photo, crib card, blanket, etc.
  - Encourage participation in support groups.
  - Provide referrals for peer counseling.
  - Provide referrals for counseling support as needed.

Appendices

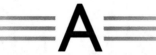

A

Immunization Schedule From Birth to 15 Months

A. IMMUNIZATION SCHEDULE FROM BIRTH TO 15 MONTHS

Immunization Schedule From Birth to 15 Months

Vaccine	Birth	1 mo	2 mos	4 mos	6 mos	9 mos	12 mos	15 mos
Hepatitis B (Hep B)	←1st dose→	←2nd dose→			←3rd dose→			
Rotavirus (RV) RV-1 (2-dose series); RV-5 (3-dose series)			←1st dose→	←2nd dose→				
Diphtheria, tetanus, and acellular pertussis (DTaP; < 7 yrs)			←1st dose→	←2nd dose→	←3rd dose→			←4th dose→
Tetanus, diphtheria, and acellular pertussis (Tdap; ≥ 7 yrs)								
Haemophilus influenzae type b (Hib)			←1st dose→	←2nd dose→			←3rd or 4th dose	
Pneumococcal conjugate (PCV13)			←1st dose→	←2nd dose→	←3rd dose→		←4th dose→	
Inactivated poliovirus (IPV; < 18 years)			←1st dose→	←2nd dose→	←3rd dose→			

(continued)

	Annual vaccination (IIV only)						
Influenza (IIV; LAIV) 2 doses for some: see footnote 8							
Measles, mumps, rubella (MMR)				←1st dose→			
Varicella (VAR)				←1st dose→			
Hepatitis A (Hep A)				←2 dose series			

Source: Centers for Disease Control and Prevention. (2013f).

A. IMMUNIZATION SCHEDULE FROM BIRTH TO 15 MONTHS

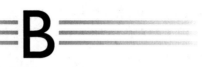

B

International Travel, Immunization, and Feeding Recommendations

RECOMMENDATIONS FOR INTERNATIONAL TRAVEL

Ideally, newborn international travel is not recommended because infants cannot be immunized prior to 6 weeks of age. Although some immunizations can be administered at 6 weeks of age, others cannot, making complete vaccination impossible in early infancy. Although aircraft travel does not pose an increased risk of infection due to air quality or recirculation of air within the air cabin in flight (Centers for Disease Control and Prevention [CDC], 2013a), prolonged flights do involve close contact with others for extended periods of time. In the event other passengers do have an infectious illness and are in close proximity to the newborn, the risk of infection would be increased in any individual with reduced immunity (including newborns). Travel precautions should include:

- Frequent handwashing or use of hand sanitizer.
- Caution is warranted when washing bottles and pacifiers to prevent contamination from unpurified water sources.

- Disinfection with cleaning agents of items that come in contact with the newborn.
- Keep infant wrapped and held if a car seat is not available.

RECOMMENDED IMMUNIZATIONS FOR INTERNATIONAL TRAVEL

Infants traveling outside of the United States are particularly vulnerable to infectious disease due to their immature immune systems and lack of adequate vaccinations resulting from their young age. International travel requires preplanning and specific interventions to ensure infant safety. Parents should be advised to:

- Consult a travel immunization specialist to determine which specific vaccines are needed for the country of travel.
- Breastfeeding women should be immunized based on recommendations for the specific travel itinerary.
- Live vaccines are safe for breastfeeding women and are not contraindicated.
- Minimal recommended vaccinations include *Haemophilus influenzae* type b (Hib); measles, mumps, rubella (MMR; CDC, 2013f).
- Specific immunizations are based on the country of travel and time of year traveling.
- Consult pediatrician 3 to 4 months ahead of travel to initiate an accelerated vaccine schedule.
- If possible, travel should be delayed until infant is 9 months of age, when yellow fever vaccine can be given.
- All infants should receive meningococcal meningitis vaccine prior to any overseas travel.
- Counsel parents that some vaccines cannot be given early.

INFANT FEEDING DURING INTERNATIONAL TRAVEL

- Breastfeeding is the safest feeding choice.
- Breastfeeding women should avoid drinking unpurified water.
- Expressed milk may be stored and transported for up to 6 to 8 hours at room temperature.
- Fresh milk may be safely stored in an insulated cooler bag with frozen ice packs for up to 24 hours.
- Refrigerated milk can be stored for 5 days.
- If refrigeration is not available and pumping is needed, milk should be discarded after 8 hours.
- If a breastfeeding mother develops "traveler's diarrhea" during international travel, more frequent breastfeeding with increased oral fluids for the mother is recommended (CDC, 2009).
- Oral rehydration salts therapy is considered safe for breastfeeding women (CDC, 2009).
- Kaolin-pectin (Kaopectate) is the antidiarrheal of choice for breastfeeding women (CDC, 2009).
- If formula is used, parents should bring formula with them and only use purified water to mix formula.

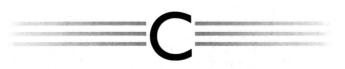

Common Abbreviations Used in Newborn Nursing

A/B—apnea/bradycardia spell (episode of apnea and/or bradycardia)

A/B/D—apnea/bradycardia/oxygen desaturation spell (episode of apnea and/or bradycardia and/or decreased oxygen saturation)

AGA—appropriate for gestational age

ARNP—advanced registered nurse practitioner (PNP or NNP)

ASD—atrial septal defect

BAT—brown adipose tissue (brown fat)

BBT—baby's blood type

BF—breastfeeding

BM—bowel movement

BPD—bronchopulmonary dysplasia

CBG—capillary blood gas

CHD—congenital heart defect or congenital heart disease

CHF—congestive heart failure

CMV—cytomegalovirus

CNM—certified nurse midwife

CNS—central nervous system

CNS—certified nurse specialist

CPAP—continuous positive airway pressure

CPT—chest physiotherapy

C/S—cesarean section

CSF—cerebrospinal fluid

CVN—central venous nutrition

CXR—chest x-ray

DIC—disseminated intravascular coagulation

DR—delivery room

EBM—expressed breast milk

ECMO—extracorporeal membrane oxygenation

ELBW—extremely low birth weight

ETC—emergency treatment center

ETT—endotracheal tube

FF—formula fed

FOC—fronto-occipital circumference

FTP—failure to progress

GBS—group B streptococcus

GDM—gestational diabetes

G-P—gravida _____ para_____ (pregnancies; pregnancies resulting in the birth after 20 weeks)

HB, HGB, Hb, or Hgb—hemoglobin

HC—head circumference

HCT—hematocrit

HFJV—high-frequency jet ventilation

HFOV—high-frequency oscillating ventilation

HFV—high-frequency ventilation

HM—human milk

HMD—hyaline membrane disease

HMF—human milk fortifier (makes breast milk 0.8 kcal/mL)

HRN—high-risk nursery

HSV—herpes simplex virus

HUS—head ultrasound

IAB or IAb—induced abortion

IDM—infant of diabetic mother

IMV—intermittent mandatory ventilation

ISAM—infant of substance-abusing mother

IU—international units

IUFD—intrauterine fetal demise

IUGR—intrauterine growth restriction

IVF—in-vitro fertilization

IVH—intraventricular hemorrhage

L & D—labor and delivery

LGA—large for gestational age

LLSB—lower left sternal border

LSB—left sternal border

MAP—mean airway pressure

MAS—meconium aspiration syndrome

MBT—mother's blood type

MCL—midclavicular line

MGF—maternal grandfather

MGM—maternal grandmother

NAD—no apparent distress

NAVA—neurally adjusted ventilatory assistance

NC—nasal cannula

NEC—necrotizing enterocolitis

NICU—neonatal intensive care unit

NNP—neonatal nurse practitioner

NNS—neonatal screen (newborn metabolic screen)

NO—nitric oxide

NP—nurse practitioner

NPCPAP—nasopharyngeal continuous positive airway
  pressure

NPO—nothing by mouth (nothing per os)

NSIMV—nasopharyngeal synchronized intermittent
  mandatory ventilation

NTD—neural tube defect

NVN—neonatal venous nutrition (local term; not
  recommended for external communication)

PC—pressure control

PCO_2—partial pressure of carbon dioxide

PCP—primary care provider

PDA—patent ductus arteriosus

PEEP—positive end- expiratory pressure

PF—premature infant formula

PFC—persistent fetal circulation

PFO—patent foramen ovale

PGE1—prostaglandin E1

PGF—paternal grandfather

PGM—paternal grandmother

PICC—percutaneously inserted central catheter

PIE—pulmonary interstitial emphysema

PIP—peak inspiratory pressure

PIV—peripheral intravenous line

PKU—phenylketonuria, a disease detected on the NNS

PMI—point of maximum impulse

PNP—pediatric nurse practitioner

PO_2—partial pressure of oxygen

PPH—persistent pulmonary hypertension

PPHN—persistent pulmonary hypertension of the newborn

PPROM—preterm premature rupture of membranes

PPS—peripheral pulmonic stenosis

PRBC—packed red blood cell (concentrated erythrocyte suspension for transfusion)

PROM—premature (before the onset of labor) or prolonged rupture of a membrane

PTD—preterm delivery

PTL—preterm labor

PVL—periventricular leukomalacia

PVN—parenteral venous nutrition or peripheral venous nutrition

RA—room air (21% oxygen)

RCM—right costal margin

RDS—respiratory distress syndrome

ROM—range of motion

ROM—rupture of membranes

ROP—retinopathy of prematurity

RSV—respiratory syncytial virus

SAB or SAb—spontaneous abortion

SF—stock formula or standard formula (iron-fortified term-infant formula)

SGA—small for gestational age

SIMV—synchronized intermittent mandatory ventilation

SO_2—oxygen saturation

STI—sexually transmitted infection

SVD—spontaneous vaginal delivery

TCM—transcutaneous monitor (for PO_2, PCO_2)

TG—true glucose (more appropriately called blood glucose; there is no "false" glucose)

TOLAC—trial of labor after cesarean

TORCH—toxoplasmosis, rubella, cytomegalovirus, herpes

TPN—total parenteral nutrition

TTN—transient tachypnea of the newborn

UAC—umbilical arterial catheter

UVC—umbilical venous catheter

VBAC—vaginal birth after cesarean

VD—vaginal delivery

VLBW—very low birth weight

VS—vital signs

VSD—ventricular septal defect

References

Adams, J. M., & Stark, A. R. (2013). Persistent pulmonary hypertension of the newborn. *Evidence-Based Clinical Decision Support at the Point of Care | UpToDate*. Retrieved October 13, 2013, from http://www.uptodate.com/contents/persistent-pulmonary-hypertension-of-the-newborn?source=search_result&selected Title=1~25

Baltimore, R. S. (2003). Neonatal sepsis. *Pediatric Drugs, 5*(11), 723–740.

Bissinger, R. L., & Annibale, D. J. (2010). Thermoregulation in very low-birth-weight infants during the golden hour: Results and implications. *Advances in Neonatal Care, 10*(5), 230–238.

Brand, P. L. (2004). What is the normal range of blood glucose concentration in healthy term newborns? *Archives of Disease in Childhood—Fetal and Neonatal Edition, 89*(4), F375–F375.

Canahuati, J. (1998). Hypoglycaemia of the newborn: Review of the literature. *Journal of Human Lactation, 14*(2), 167–168.

Centers for Disease Control and Prevention. (2009). *Food-borne and waterborne illness.* Retrieved from http://www.cdc.gov/breastfeeding/disease/food_illness.htmnter

Centers for Disease Control and Prevention. (2012). *Fetal alcohol spectrum disorders.* Retrieved from http://www.cdc.gov/ncbddd/fasd/index.html

Centers for Disease Control and Prevention. (2013a). *Air travel.* Retrieved from http://wwwnc.cdc.gov/travel/yellowbook/2014/chapter-6-conveyance-and-transportation-issues/air-travel

Centers for Disease Control and Prevention. (2013b). *Birth defects.* Retrieved from http://www.cdc.gov/ncbddd/birthdefects/data.html

Centers for Disease Control and Prevention. (2013c). *Facts about congenital heart defects.* Retrieved from http://www.cdc.gov/ncbddd/heartdefects/hlhs.html

Centers for Disease Control and Prevention. (2013d). *State vaccination requirements.* Retrieved from http://www.cdc.gov/vaccines/imz-managers/laws/index.html

Centers for Disease Control and Prevention. (2013e). *Sudden unexpected infant death and sudden infant death syndrome.* Retrieved from http://www.cdc.gov/sids

Centers for Disease Control and Prevention. (2013f). *Vaccine recommendations for infants & children.* Retrieved from http://wwwnc.cdc.gov/travel/yellowbook/2014/chapter-7-international-travel-infants-children/vaccine-recommendations-for-infants-and-children

Congenital and Children's Heart Center. (2013). *Selected heart conditions.* Retrieved from http://www.childrensheartcentre.com/index.html

Courtwright, A. M., Laughon, M. M., & Doron, M. W. (2011). Length of life and treatment intensity in infants diagnosed prenatally or postnatally with congenital anomalies considered to be lethal. *Journal of Perinatology, 31*(6), 387–391.

Davidson, M. R., London, M. L., & Ladewig, P. W. (2011). *Old's maternal–newborn nursing & women's health across the lifespan* (9th ed.). Boston: Pearson.

Devereux, G., McNeill, G., Newman, G., Turner, S., Craig, L., Martindale, S., . . ., Seaton, A. (2007). Early childhood wheezing symptoms in relation to plasma selenium in pregnant mothers and neonates. *Clinical & Experimental Allergy, 37*(7), 1000–1008.

Guglani, L., Lakshminrusimha, S., & Ryan, R. M. (2008). Transient tachypnea of the newborn. *Pediatrics in Review, 29*(11), e59–e65.

Harrington, J. W. (2011). Vaccination refusal: How to counsel the vaccine-hesitant parent. *Consultant for Pediatricians, 10*(11), 321–328.

Hillman, N. (2007). Hyperbilirubinemia in the late preterm infant. *Newborn and Infant Nursing Reviews, 7*(2), 91–94.

Lemons, J. A., Bauer, C. R., Oh, W., Korones, S. B., Papile, L. A., & Stoll, B. J. (2001). Very low birth weight outcomes of the National Institute of Child Health and Human Development

Neonatal Research Network, January 1995 through December 1996. NICHD Neonatal Research Network. *Pediatrics, 107,* E1.

National Institutes of Health: AIDS Information. (2012). *Recommendations for use of antiretroviral drugs in pregnant HIV-1-infected women for maternal health and interventions to reduce perinatal HIV transmission in the United States.* Retrieved from http://aidsinfo.nih.gov/guidelines/html/3/perinatal-guidelines/188

Persson, B. (2009). Neonatal glucose metabolism in offspring of mothers with varying degrees of hyperglycemia during pregnancy. *Seminars in Fetal and Neonatal Medicine, 14*(2), 106–110.

Pettersen, M. D., & Niash, S. R. (2013). Pediatric complete atrioventricular septal defects follow-up. *Medscape.* Retrieved from http://emedicine.medscape.com/article/893914-followup#a2650

Verani, J. R., McGee, L., & Schrag, S. J. (2010). *Prevention of perinatal group B streptococcal disease: Revised guidelines from CDC, 2010.* Atlanta, GA: Department of Health and Human Services, Centers for Disease Control and Prevention.

Wainer, S., Rabi, J., & Lyon, M. (2007). Coombs' testing and neonatal hyperbilirubinemia. *Canadian Medical Association Journal, 176*(7), 972–973.

Winn, H. (2007). Group B streptococcus infection in pregnancy. *Clinics in Perinatology, 34*(3), 387–392.

Woods, D. (2012, August 12). Management of the infant with asphyxia. *Geneva Foundation for Medical Education and Research.* Retrieved October 13, 2013, from http://www.gfmer.ch/PEP/Asphyxia.htm

Index